The DIETER'S ALMANAC

A Full Year's Guide to Weight Loss
and Body Firmness

Theodore Berland

World Almanac Publications
New York, New York

ABOUT THE AUTHOR

Theodore Berland is author of 14 books, including *The Fitness Fact Book*, *Rating the Diets*, and *The Doctor's Calories-Plus Diet*. He is associated with Michael Reese Hospital and Medical Center, Chicago, and Grand Valley State College, Allendale, Michigan. At a height of 5 feet 11 inches, he weighs 153 pounds. Several times each week, year-round, he jogs five miles and swims one.

Illustrations: Jeanette Eng-Hom
Design: Thomas P. Ruis

First published in 1984.

Distributed in the United States by Ballantine Books, a division of Random House, Inc., and in Canada by Random House of Canada, Ltd.

Library of Congress Catalog Card Number: 83-051724
Newspaper Enterprise Association ISBN: 0-91181-48-0
Ballantine Books ISBN: 0-345-31628-2

Printed in the United States of America

World Almanac Publications
Newspaper Enterprise Association, Inc.
A division of United Media Enterprises
A Scipps-Howard company
200 Park Avenue
New York, NY 10166

For Frieda, my other mother

Also by Theodore Berland

The Scientific Life
Your Children's Teeth
Living With Your Ulcer
Living With Your Bad Back
Living With Your Bronchitis and Emphysema
Living With Your Eye Operation
Living With Your Colitis and Hemorrhoids and Related Disorders
Rating the Diets (Diets '74-'83)
The Acupuncture Diet
After the Diet. . . Then What?
The Fitness Fact Book
The Doctor's Calories-Plus Diet
Living With Your Allergies and Asthma

CONTENTS

INTRODUCTION

Dieting is an everyday, every week, year-round activity. Successful dieters know that weight can be lost and kept off only if they work at it constantly. Those wonderfully lean bodies you admire belong to persons who constantly attend to their physical fitness.

The slim and the muscular are not supermen or superwomen; they are just like you. The difference between you and them is that they have made fitness and weight control important parts of their life. If you want to be like them, so must you. This means including diet and exercise in your daily activities and your weekly thoughts in every season, year in and year out.

Weight control cannot take a holiday because weight gain never goes. But don't misconstrue. This does not mean that dieting and exercise have to be drudgery. They can be fun activities, a game of life. But, as in playing any game, you need to have your mind on it, you need to be aware of what is going on, and you need to be always conscious of the presence of your opponents: appetite and sluggishness.

The Dieter's Almanac is here to help you win, to help you lose weight and keep it off, and to be firm. It can help you understand your feelings about food, your emotional investment in food, your bad eating habits, and your seasonal eating cycles. It offers information on good foods to eat, bad foods to avoid, and the truths about both effective and foolish diets. There is also information here about exercising in the four seasons. A 90-day exercise program is offered; it will make you firmer, harder, stronger, and more enduring.

The Dieter's Almanac is a book to keep close to you. It should be your companion, your daily guide, your source of accurate and useful information, your occasional inspiration when your spirits are low, and your gentle reminder when you temporarily go off your diet or exercise program.

There should be no need to sell you on the importance of diet and exercise. That's why you have picked up and are now reading *The Dieter's Almanac*. Still, here is some information to reinforce your resolve to lose weight and gain firmness.

1. A 1979 report on a survey by the U.S. Department of Agriculture revealed that although American men and women ate fewer calories but more fats in the 1970s than they did in the 1960s, their average weight did not drop. Dr. D. Mark Hegsted, administrator of the USDA's Human Nutrition Center, observed, "We are as big and fat as we ever were and obesity may be gaining on us. About the only interpretation possible at this time would be that Americans are becoming increasingly sedentary."
2. Two government surveys published by the National Center for Health Statistics indicated that Americans are constantly gaining weight: Men 3 pounds, women 1 pound, on the average, in 10 years. Women who were 5 feet 4 inches tall and 18 to

44 years old gained the most: 4 to 7 pounds, on the average, during the decade between the surveys.

3. Another U.S. government study, conducted from 1976 through 1980, found that one in six men and one in four women weigh 20 percent more than the average. Moreover, one in three men and two in three women in America are 10 percent overweight.

Millions of overweight people, in their desperation to lose weight, swallow the baloney of diet hucksters. A 1981 editorial in *Obesity/Bariatric Medicine* observed the overabundance of "unregulated . . . self-styled 'nutritionists,' 'diet experts,' and purveyors of quack remedies and devices ready to prey upon an overweight public. . . . The hype surrounding these allegedly effective therapies includes media quackery made to appear credible by so-called 'experts' on the ubiquitous TV talk shows, or through blatant touting in tabloids found at supermarkets or newsstands." The information marketplace is flooded with "myths, misconceptions, and half-truths involving diets and nutrition."

A 1982 survey made by dietitian Marsha Hudnall for the American Council on Science and Health in New York City confirmed those observations. She carefully studied and evaluated the information about nutrition offered in 19 major magazines and found that only five (*50 Plus, Parents, Redbook, Reader's Digest*, and *Good Housekeeping*) published "generally reliable" information. Eight others contained mixtures of valid and invalid information, and six magazines were consistent sources of unreliable information about nutrition.

Thus, in an era of information abundance, many (or most) people who want to lose weight are receiving misinformation. As sophisticated as we are, in this second-to-last decade before the 21st century, we are suckers for the nonsense sold by fast-buck diet hucksters.

With *The Dieter's Almanac*, you can close your ears to the hucksters' sweet talk and live an easy-to-follow, week-by-week program of simple, effective dieting and exercise. *The Dieter's Almanac* is a book to live with and live by. It is honest, it is forthright, it is revealing, and it is insightful. Most of all, it is useful. It is crammed with facts and figures, with solid information you can use to lose weight and make yourself slim and firm. It doesn't preach, yet it offers solid advice. It is not rigid, yet it follows the highest standards of nutrition and physical training. It offers one year's worth of programs, yet it can be used perennially.

If you need motivation to shape up, look at the following list of 41 good reasons to begin a fitness program. They are disorders linked to overweight, compiled by Dr. Theodore B. Van Italie of St. Luke's Hospital Center, New York City, and published in The *American Journal of Clinical Nutrition*. You can avoid most or all of these ailments by getting down to proper weight and staying there.

Heart: premature coronary heart disease, left ventricular hypertrophy, angina pectoris, sudden death (ventricular arrhythmia), congestive heart failure.

Vascular system: hypertension, stroke (cerebral infarction, hemorrhage, or both), venous stasis with lower extremity edema, varicose veins, hemorrhoids, thromboembolic disease (involving lower extremities and inferior vena cava).

Respiratory system: obstructive sleep apnea, Pickwickian syndrome (alveola hypoventilation), secondary polycythemia, right ventricular hypertrophy (sometimes leading to failure).

Hepatobiliary system: choleithiasis, hepatic steatosis, hormonal and metabolic functions, diabetes mellitus (insulin independent), gout (hyperuricemia), hyperlipidemias (hypertriglyceridemia and hypercholesterolemia).

Kidney: proteinuria and (in very severe obesity) nephrosis, renal vein thrombosis.

Skin: striae, acanthosis nigricans (benign type), hirsutism, intertrigo, plantar callus, multiple papillomas.

Joints, muscles, and connective tissue: osteoarthritis of knees, bone spurs of the heel, osteoarthrosis of spine (in women), aggravation of preexisting postural faults.

Neoplasia: increased risk of endometrial cancer, possible increased risk of breast cancer.

Reproductive and sexual function: impaired obstetrical performance (increased risk of toxemia, hypertension, and diabetes mellitus during pregnancy, prolonged labor, more frequent need for caesarian section), irregular menstruation and frequent anovulatory cycles, reduced fertility.

Psychosocial function: impairment of self-image with feelings of inferiority; social isolation; subject to social, economic and other kinds of discrimination; susceptibility to psychoneuroses; loss of mobility; increased employee absenteeism.

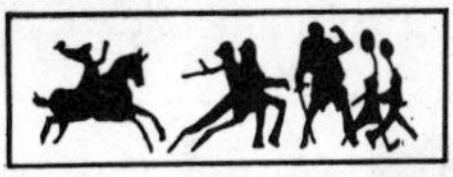

HOW TO USE THIS ALMANAC

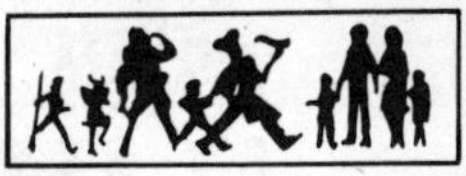

The Dieter's Almanac is arranged by week so that you can concentrate on a different theme for every one of the 52 weeks in the year. There is no repetitive pattern because that would bore you. There are themes, however, including which foods to eat and not eat, praise for good diets to follow and warnings about diets not to follow, and how to get in shape and stay that way.

As you might expect, *The Dieter's Almanac* emphasizes seasons and holidays. This not only gives you renewed inspiration and motivation but also helps prepare you to get the best out of this season and get ready for the next season. Proper preparation is never so important in human activities as it is in tasks that require effort—tasks like dieting and exercise. Half the success of winning a battle is being ready for it. *The Dieter's Almanac* helps you get ready not only for fighting the battle, but for winning it!

Still, there may be days when you are interested in a specific subject. No, it isn't cheating to turn to another part of *The Dieter's Almanac* in order to get information on a topic not scheduled for this week. Keep in mind that *The Dieter's Almanac* is here to serve you, to help you get slim and firm.

The Dieter's Almanac can serve you in many ways. Use it as you wish. What's important is that you do use it, that it helps you to help yourself.

THE DIETER'S ALMANAC EXERCISE PLAN

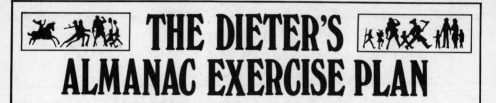

This exercise plan is not for marathon runners, speed swimmers, gymnasts, or champion cyclists. It is for you. It is a safe and effective way to slim down, toughen up, and stay that way.

The exercises are programmed so as to ease you into, and hold you at, four levels of tough slimness:

1. Flexibility
2. Firmness
3. Strength
4. Endurance

The Dieter's Almanac Exercise Plan begins mildly on New Year's Day and becomes slightly more rigorous at every new stage. The slow progression is designed to make your body more supple—gently; to make your muscles firmer and stronger—without bulging; and to enable you to exercise longer and harder—*without gasping and pain.*

The *Almanac*'s exercise program requires three months to get you to top fitness and firmness. Then, by following the maintenance exercise program, you can stay at your peak for the rest of the year and for years to come.

You start the program with flexibility exercises, which soon become your daily warmup exercises. This is the stretching regime you will do before starting any and every activity.

Then you add a second kind of exercise, one that will firm the fat out of your muscles.

The third level of exercising is designed to strengthen your muscles.

The fourth level consists of physical activities that will extend your ability to exercise vigorously. By this time you will be able to jog, fast-walk, swim, climb stairs, or cycle without losing your wind and without feeling your heart pounding in your throat.

A few words about spot-reducing exercises: They work, but only if you know how to use them. To reduce fat, you have to actively exercise the muscles in the area you want lean. That means exercising every day. Repetition keeps muscles lean. (Repetitive exercises cannot help lean down nonmuscular areas which accumulate fat, such as breasts or chin.)

To lean down a muscle area, you don't need to exert as much force as you do to strengthen a muscle. Muscle building requires lots of effort in a short burst of time. Then you need to rest, to allow the muscle to recover and build new fibers. So muscle building is best accomplished by exercising every other day.

Your exercise program should include all four exercise levels. Your eventual goal should be: 5 minutes of flexibility and warmup exercises, 10 minutes of strengthening and slimming exercises, and 30 minutes of endurance activities.

You'll find that the day after you do a new stretch or add more exercises you'll be sore and perhaps a bit stiff. Work those sore muscles carefully, but do work them. Remember: The more you do, the more you'll be able to do, and the less sore you'll be.

The same applies to your wind. You'll find you will be less and less winded as you increase your endurance activities.

Don't be too ambitious at the outset. It can lead to discouragement and then you'll quit. Be patient. Start with the Main Street Stroll the first day and add an exercise every day. Thus, on the second day you are doing Exercises 1 and 2; the third day, Exercises 1, 2, and 3, and so forth.

Outline of The Dieter's Almanac Exercise Plan

January 1-10: 10 flexibility exercises (one new one a day)
January 11-20: 10 firming exercises (one new one a day)
January 21-29: 5 strengthening exercises (one new one every other day)
January 30-February 3: 5 more flexibility exercises (one new one a day)
February 4-17: 10 minutes of endurance activity
February 18-March 3: 15 minutes of endurance activity

March 4-17: 20 minutes of endurance activity
March 18-31: 30 minutes of endurance activity

Level 1: Flexibility

Workouts are a three-act performance.
Act 1 is the warmup.
Act 2 is strenuous activity.
Act 3 is the cool-down.

Muscles and joints that are worked without warming up are prone to pain and injury. Muscle fibers that are not ready to work are easily torn. Moreover, a warmed muscle works better than a cold one. It is stronger and more responsive. And it relaxes better between efforts; that means it recovers better.

Many newcomers to exercise don't realize that the stretch is one of the more important parts of the warmup.

Stretching is important for people of all ages, but it becomes even more important as you get older. That's because ligaments, tendons, and other connective tissue involved in muscles, bones, and joints lose flexibility and elasticity with the years. Also, many middle-aged people have less fluid immediately available to lubricate their joints than they had when they were younger.

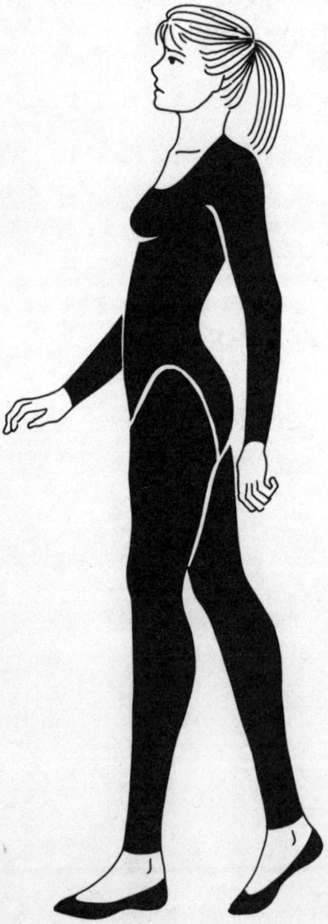

1. The Main Street Stroll: Walk around for 30 seconds with an exaggerated swing of your arms forward and backward.

2. Walk and Twist: Walk for 30 seconds, moving your arms as though you were swimming the crawl. For 15 seconds longer, clasp your hands behind your head and exaggerate the torso's twisting action as you walk.

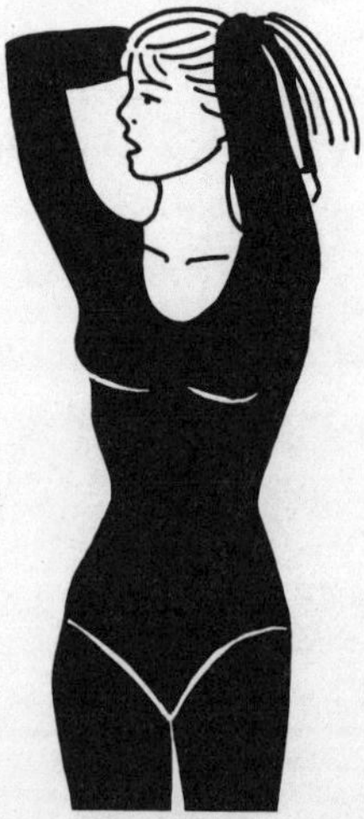

You have big joints, such as the shoulder, elbow, hip, and knee, and small joints, such as those in your fingers and toes. Your spine is also made up of joints. Many people precipitate bad backs during exercise by not prelubricating their vertebrae and warming up the muscles and tendons that hold this pile of bones vertical.

A caution: You can defeat your purpose by being too enthusiastic and overstretching a muscle during warmup. That is because muscle has a "stretch reflex." When a muscle is overstretched, it responds by contracting. This pulling-against-you reflex prevents proper muscle lengthening and can lead to soreness and even muscle strain.

The wrong way to stretch is by bouncing and bobbing. The right way to stretch is slowly and gently.

Bend, push, or pull one segment of your body at a time until you just s-t-r-e-t-c-h. Hold the position for 5 to 30 seconds. The bigger the muscle, the longer you should hold the stretch.

Your *Dieter's Almanac* shape-up program begins with flexibility exercises designed to warm you up and help you overcome the stiffness that inactivity has imposed on your muscles and joints.

Here they are:

3. Neck-Roll: Assume a standing position. Slowly roll your neck and head through the entire range of motion. Roll the head in a clockwise direction several times and then repeat in the same manner in a counterclockwise direction. Really try to loosen up the neck and shoulders as you roll. Do this 30 seconds in each direction.

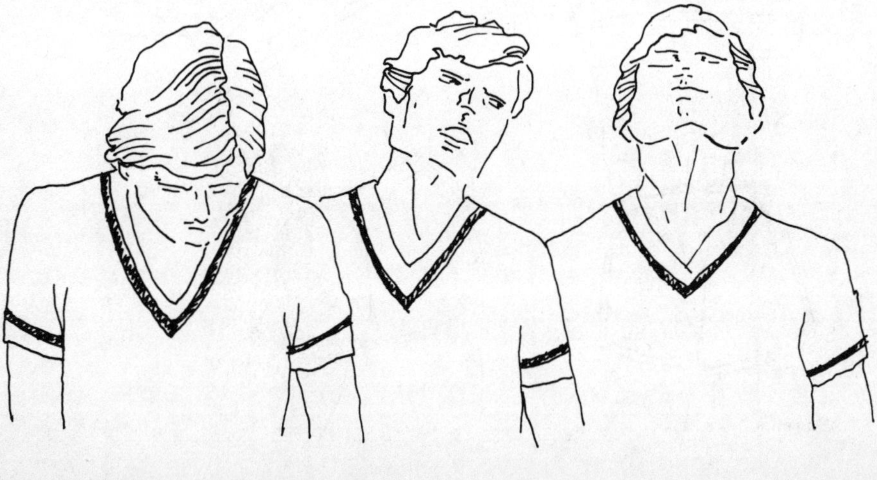

4. Lateral Side Bending: Starting from a standing position, with your hands clasped high above your head, slowly bend laterally down to the right at the waist. Hold this bent position for five to eight counts and then slowly return to the left. Repeat the lateral side bend three times for each side.

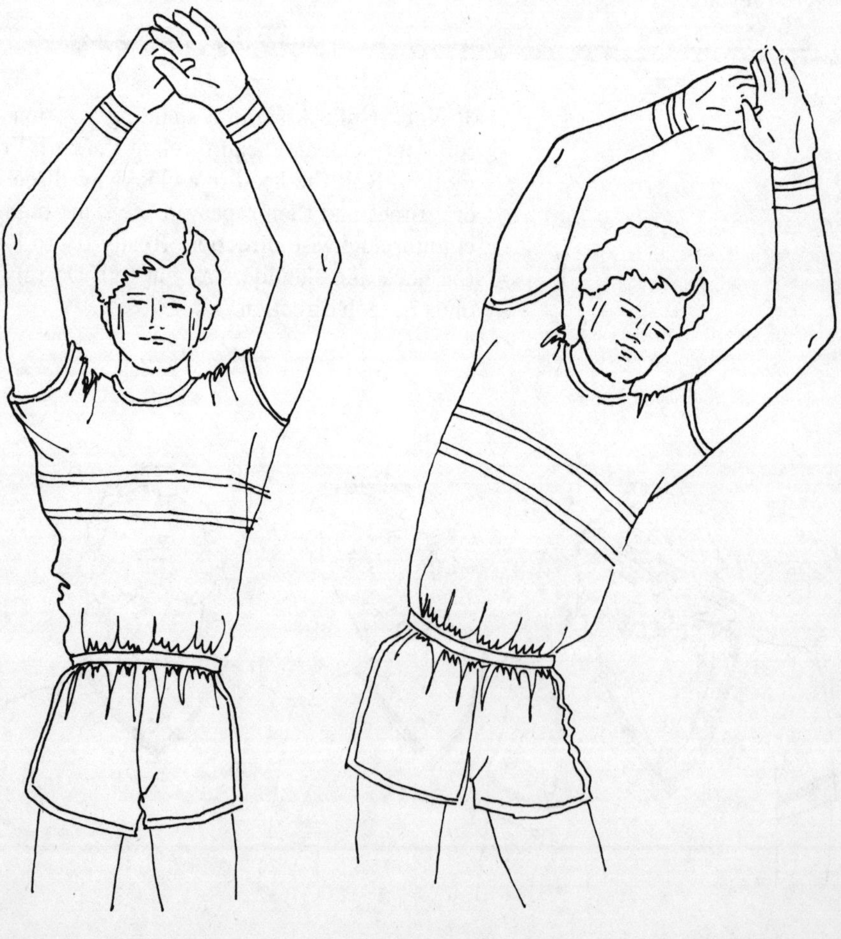

5. Alternate Floor Touch: Remain in the standing position with your feet apart. Bend forward at the waist. Place one hand down toward the floor between your feet and the other in the air above your head. Remain in this position and rotate your shoulders back and forth as you alternate touching the floor with each hand. Stay relaxed and do not bounce during this exercise. Reach toward the floor 10 times with each hand.

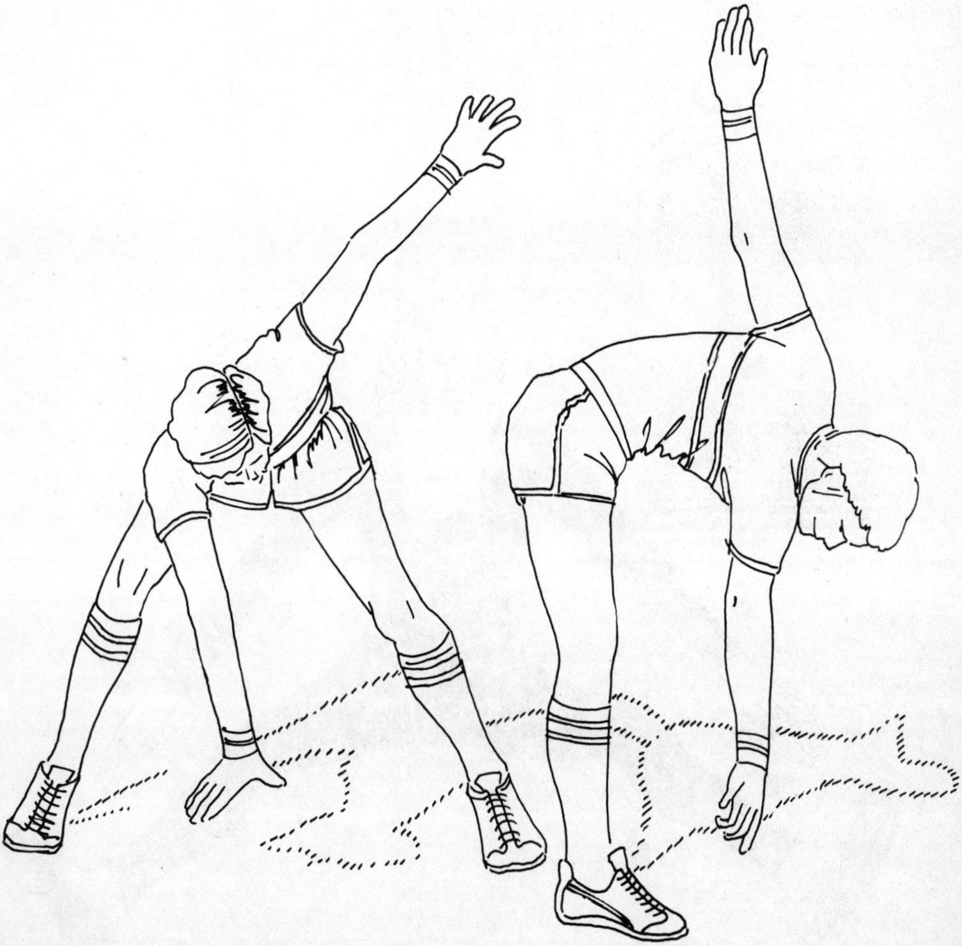

6. Sitting Stretch: This is excellent for the back of your legs and your back. Sit erect with legs apart. Bend at the waist and move your hands as far forward as possible over your legs. Eventually you'll be able to grasp your ankles with your hands. Hold 5 seconds and repeat three times.

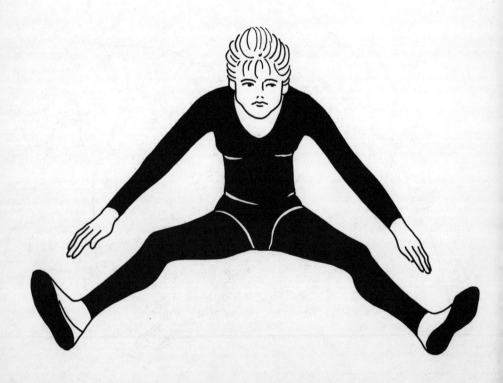

7. Hamstring Stretch: Lie on your back with your knees flexed. Raise one leg up toward the ceiling and slowly attempt to straighten it. Do not jerk or bounce. For more of a stretch, slowly push your heel up toward the ceiling. Return this leg to the flexed starting position and repeat the exercise with the other leg. Stretch five times with each leg.

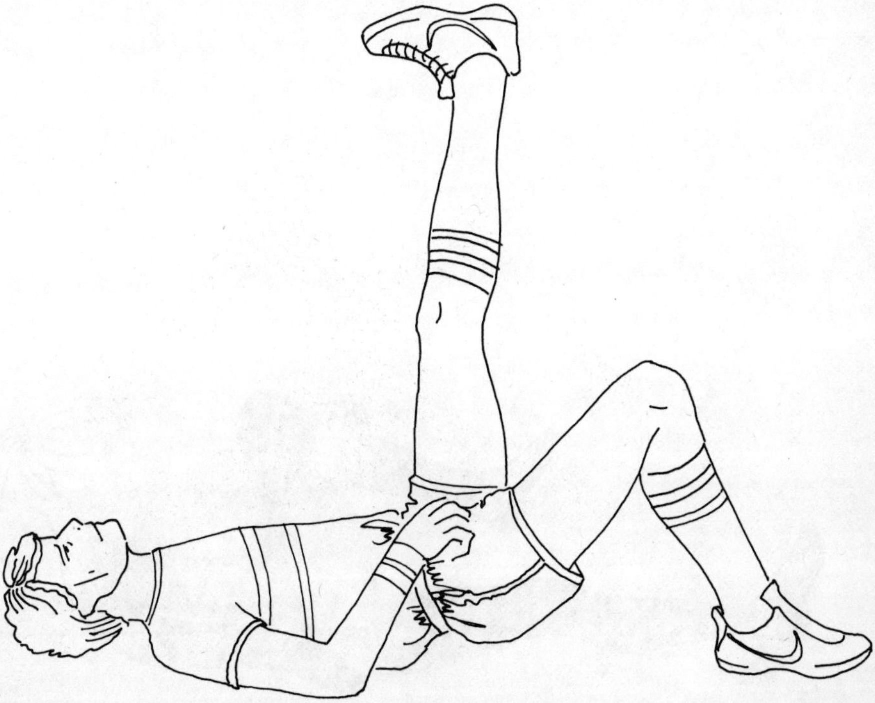

8. Knee Hugs: Lying on your back, bend one knee up. Grab it with your hands and press it gently to your chest. Then let the knee return to the floor. Repeat with the other knee. Raise each knee five times.

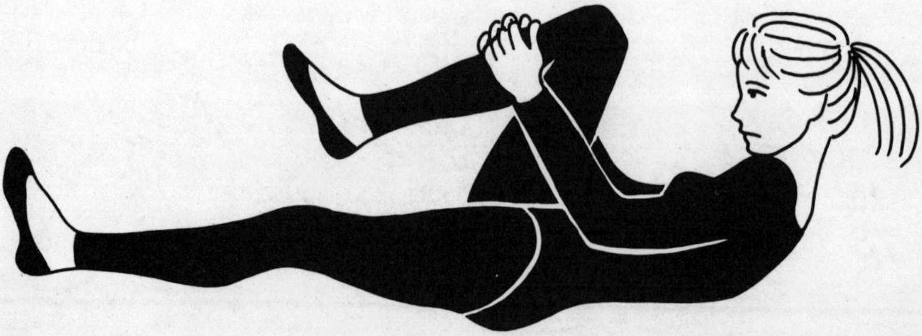

9. Side Leg Raises: Roll onto your left side. Lift and lower your right leg five times. Roll over and repeat five times with your left leg.

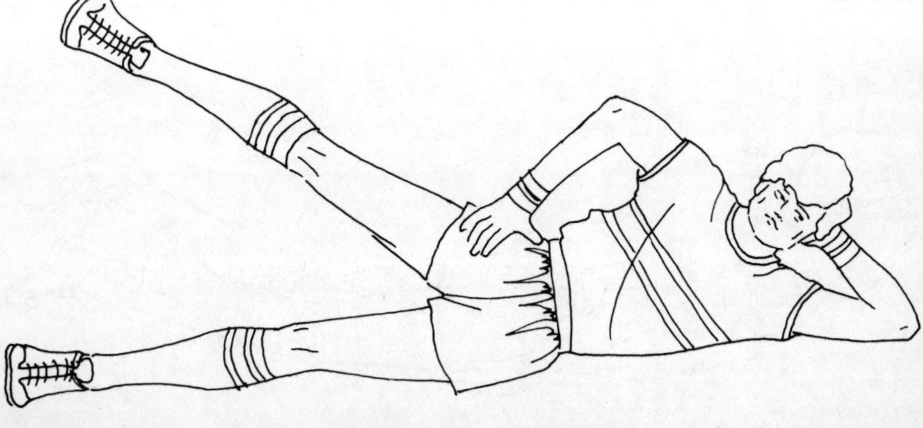

10. Flutter Kick: Lying prone with your arms at your sides, lift your legs off the floor and flutter kick for 30 seconds.

Don't rush. Take your time. Add one exercise a day until you are doing all 10 flexibility exercises every day. After 10 days, on January 11, go on to exercise Level 2.

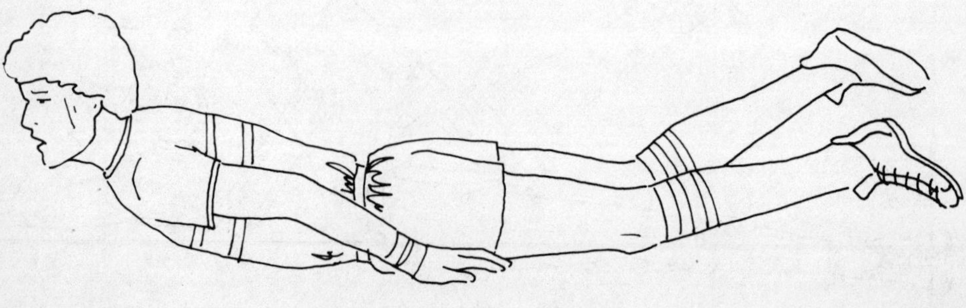

Level 2: Firmness

If you are like most people, you want some parts of your body leaner than others. Particularly, you want a flat tummy, firm thighs and derriere, and lean upper arms. At the same time, you want a full chest.

Level 2 exercises are designed to start you on the road to leanness.

First do the flexibility exercises. Then do the 10 firming exercises that follow. If your muscles feel a little sore, that's OK. It is your body's way of telling you that suppleness is coming back.

Keep in mind that you are going to have to exert yourself. Firmness doesn't just happen. You have to work for it. But it is worth the effort.

After the flexibility exercises, do five firmness exercises for the tummy. Here they are:

1. Head Raises: Lie supine with your back on the floor, your knees bent, and your feet flat. Place your hands behind your head. Tense your abdominal muscles as you lift your head toward your knees.

Be sure you don't use your hands or arms to raise your head. Let the effort come from your tummy. Don't force it. Don't try to touch your knees; just lift your head and shoulders. Repeat three times.

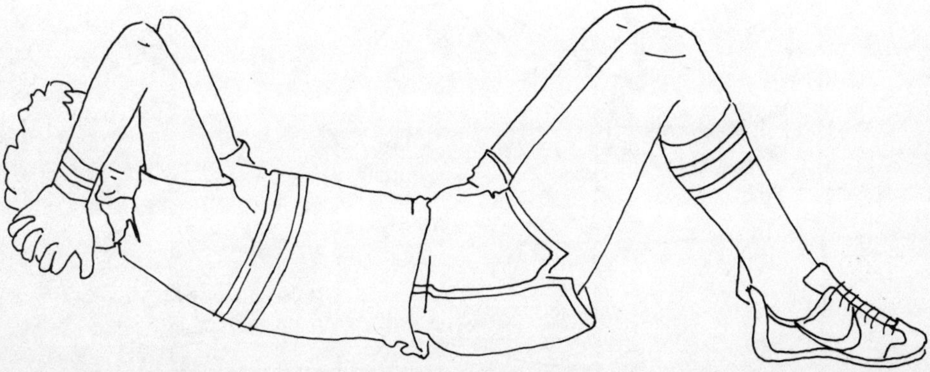

2. Roll-Ups: Begin with your back on the floor, your knees bent, and your hands behind your head. Use your abdominal muscles to roll forward and raise your torso until your head touches your knees. If you are stiff at first, go only as far as you can. Again, don't force it. It helps to place your feet under a piece of heavy furniture. Exhale as you rise; inhale as you lower yourself. Repeat three times.

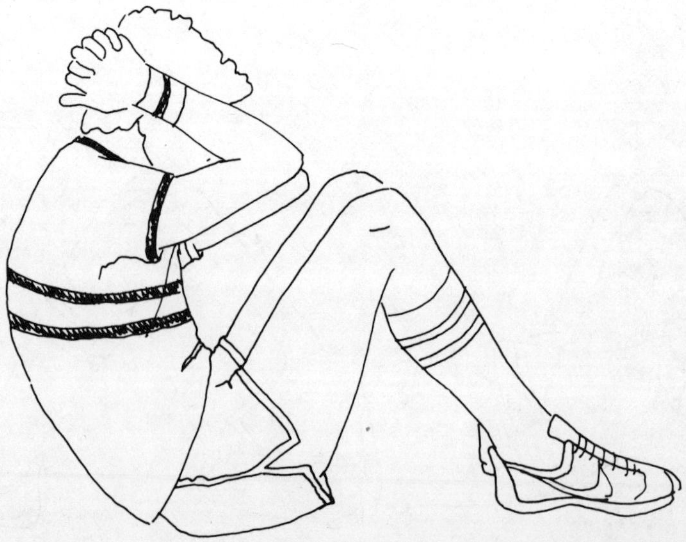

3. Leg Raises: Lie supine with your arms and legs completely extended. Your legs are stretched straight so that your heels are on the floor with your feet together. Your arms are extended above your head and are flat on the floor.

Relax a moment. Take a deep breath. Keeping both legs together, raise them until they are vertical. Keep pulling until your legs are facing you. Try to touch your fingertips with your toes. (After you have done the exercise for a while, your toes will be able to touch the floor beyond your fingertips.)

Slowly return your legs to the vertical position and slowly lower them to the floor. Repeat 10 times.

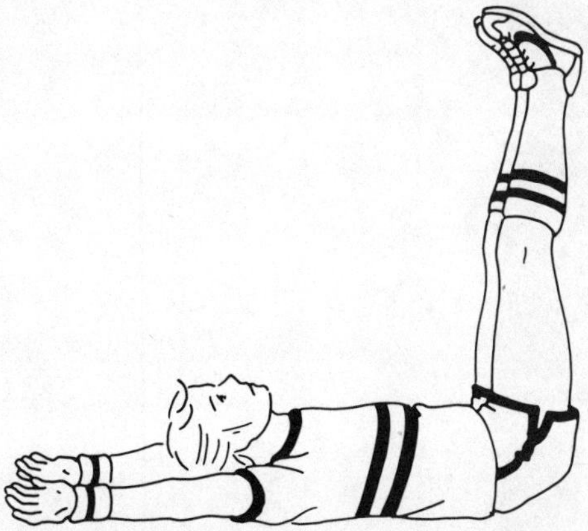

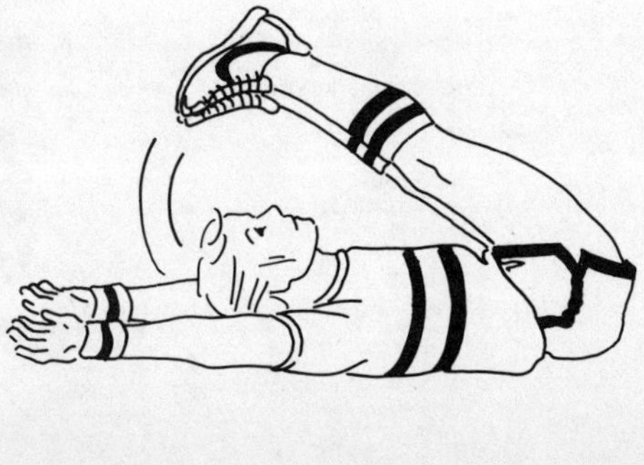

4. Lean and Bend: Stand with your back to a wall about a foot or so away. Your feet are slightly separated. Stretch your arms above your head. Slowly lean back bending at the waist, until your hands touch the wall. Keep your elbows and knees straight.

Now pull forward and drop your arms. Bend over and touch your fingers to your ankles, feet, or toes, whichever you can reach. But don't force it. Return to a standing position. Repeat five times.

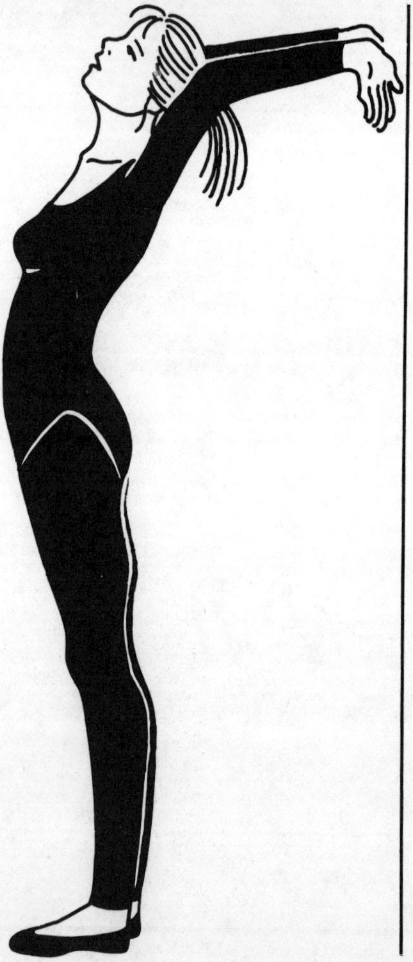

5. Isometrics: Expand your chest and pull in your tummy. Tightly. Try to suck it back against your spine. Hold for a count of six, then relax. Now push out so that you have a belly. Hold for a count of six. Relax. Exhale.

Do five sets of this exercise several times during the day. Do it in your car every time you have to stop for a signal or light. Or do it whenever you get a phone call.

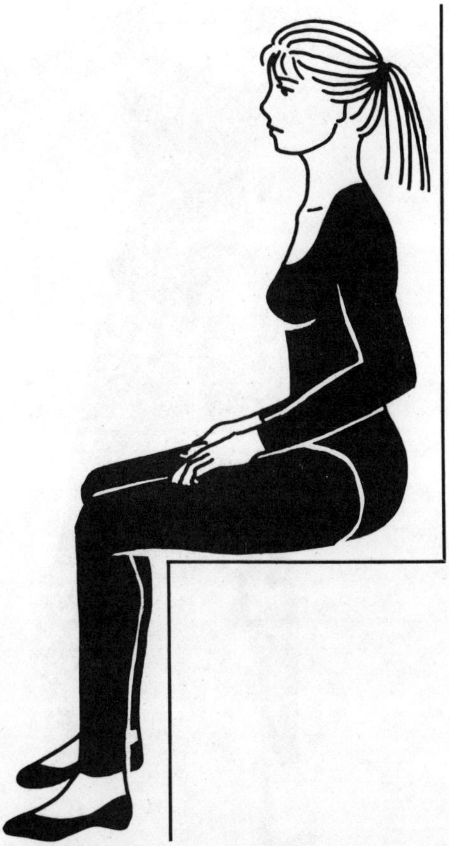

Here are two firmness exercises for your chest:

6. Samson Door Press: Standing in an open doorway with your feet apart, lift your arms until your hands are at shoulder height. Place your hands on opposite jambs of the door frame. Push out. Pretend you are Samson pushing over the pillars at the Gates of Gaza. Hold for a count of six. Repeat 10 times.

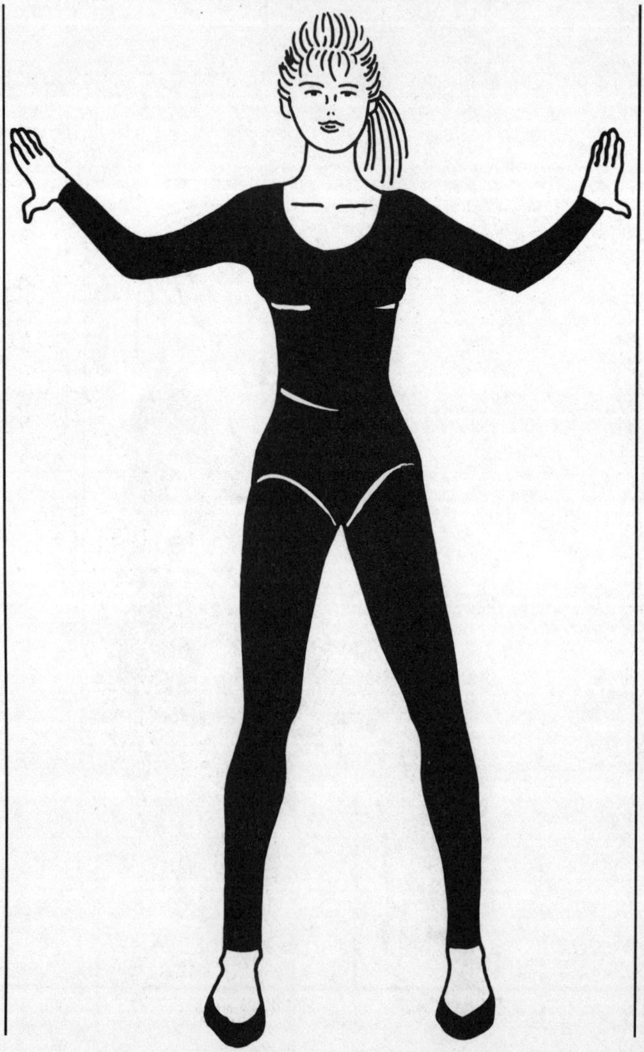

7. Wall-Push: Standing at arm's length from a wall, extend your arms forward with your palms touching the wall. Lean forward all the way. Then push back.
Do five times.

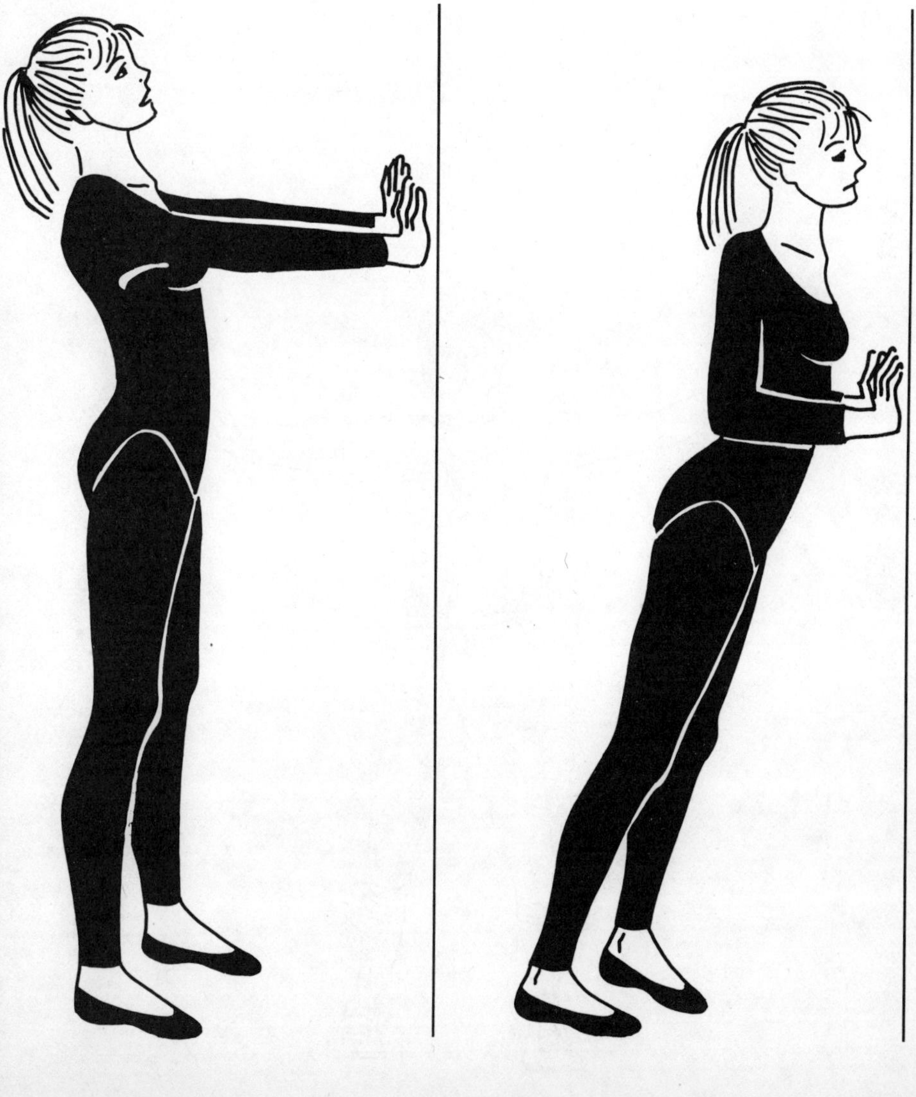

Here is one for the upper arms:

8. Arm Circles: Standing with your legs apart, extend your arms to the side with your elbows straight. With your palms up, rotate your arms so that your hands describe circles in the air. Rotate five times backward. Then turn your palms down and rotate five times forward.

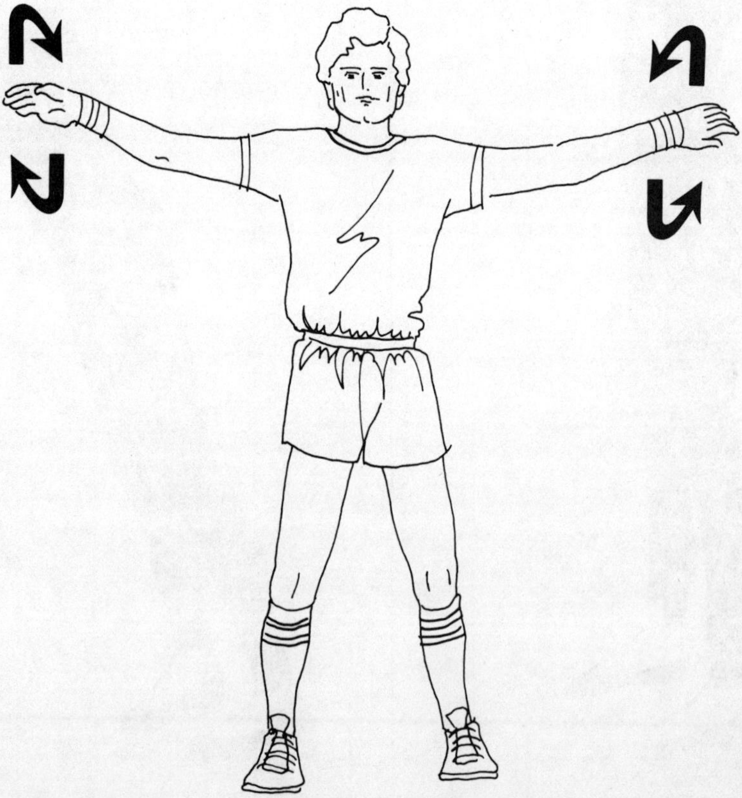

Here are two for your hips and thighs:

9. Hip Rolls: Lie on your back with your arms extended to your sides and your palms flat on the floor. Pull your legs up until your knees are over your stomach. Keeping your knees together, roll first to one side and then to the other. Do five side-to-side repetitions.

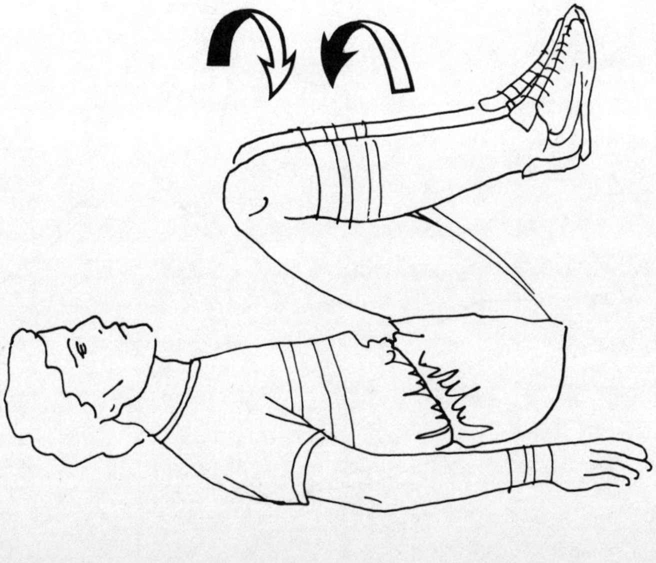

10. Thigh Slimmer: Sitting on the floor with your legs spread, lean back with your palms on the floor and your elbows straight. Pull in your tummy. Flex your right foot and raise your right leg with the knee stiff. Hold it about a foot above the floor for a count of 10. Then lower it. Repeat with the left leg. Five repetitions per leg.

If you started, *The Dieter's Almanac* Exercise Plan on January 1, and have been adding one exercise a day, you should be doing all 20 flexibility and firmness exercises by January 20. If that is where you are, you can (and should) go on to the strengthening exercises at Level 3.

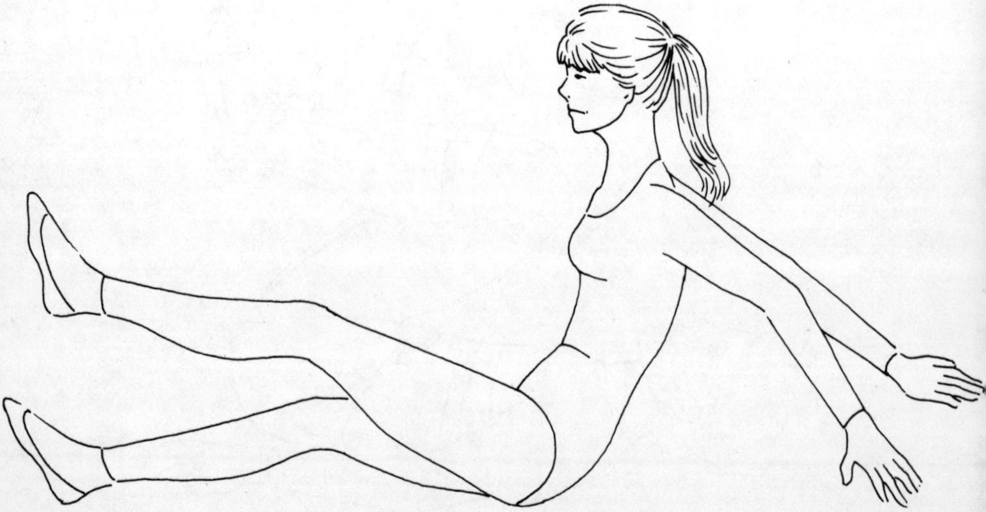

Level 3: Strength

Muscle-strengthening exercises need to be done every other day. To gain strength, muscles have to rest between exertions. Heavy exercise challenges a muscle. It requires a day or two in order to build up its strength. After that, it can meet the challenge. Repeat the challenge, and the muscle will maintain the strength necessary to meet it. Increase the challenge, as with weights, and the muscle will grow even stronger.

Unless you want your muscles to grow bulky, you need to limit the demand. You can prevent bulkiness by maintaining the same level of exercise intensity needed to keep that muscle as strong as you want it to be. And stay away from barbells.

So, starting January 21, add the first strengthening exercise. Skip a day, and on January 23, add the second strengthener. And so forth adding a new exercise on January 25, January 27, and January 29.

Here are the exercises for strengthening:

1. Shoulder Squeeze: Swing your arms across the front of your chest and around the sides as far back as possible. Grasp your shoulders with the hands as if trying to force the shoulder joints together in front. Swing the arms forward again and repeat. This exercise strengthens the upper back muscles and shoulder girdle. Repeat five times.

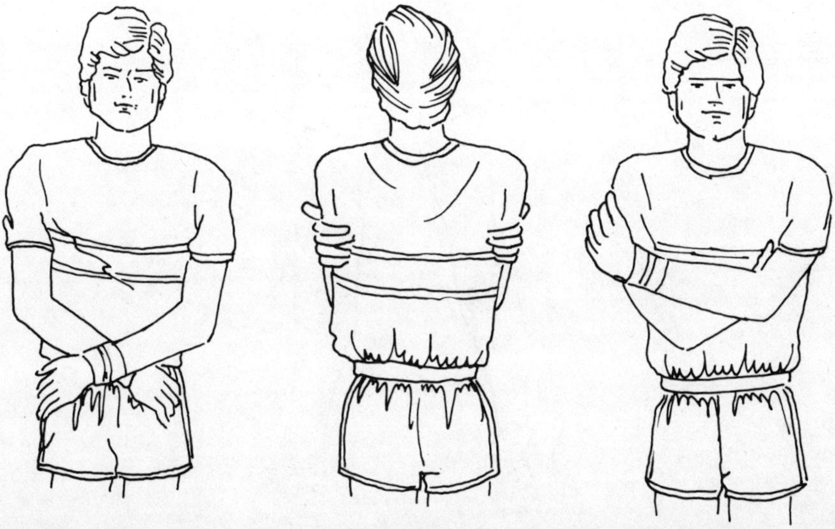

2. Chest Press-Pull: Stand with feet shoulder-width apart and hands together in front of chest, elbows held at shoulder height. Then raise arms outward and upward while inhaling. Push palms against each other. Harder, harder. Exhale as you push. Hold for count of five. Now lock fingers and try to pull apart. Harder. Harder, for a count of five. Repeat five times pushing and pulling.

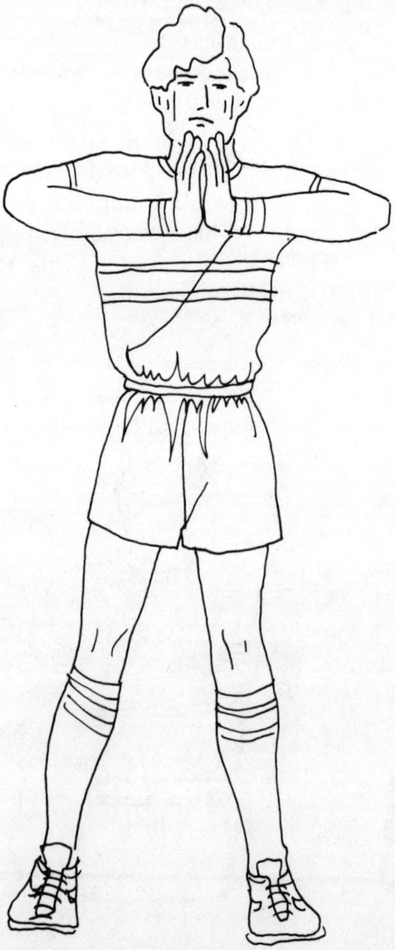

3. Squat: Begin by standing with your arms extended in front of you (or with your hands on your hips). Squat slowly until your thighs are parallel to the floor, or until your buttocks almost touch the seat of a chair. *Slowly* rise again until you are standing. Do five times.

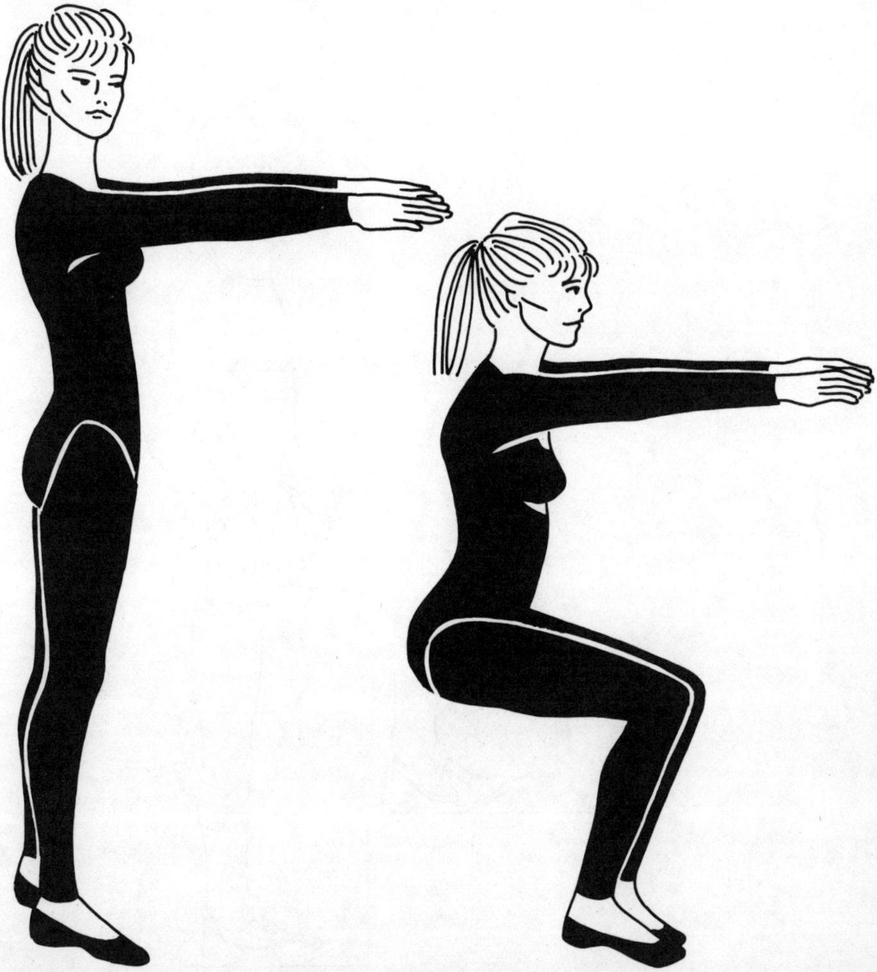

4. Step-Ups: A small step stool is all that's needed; if that's not available, simply use the nearest stairway. Start by putting your left foot on the stool (or step), then bring your right foot up. Next, return the left foot to the floor and then the right foot. The object is to get a steady 1-2-3-4 rhythm established. Do for 5 minutes.

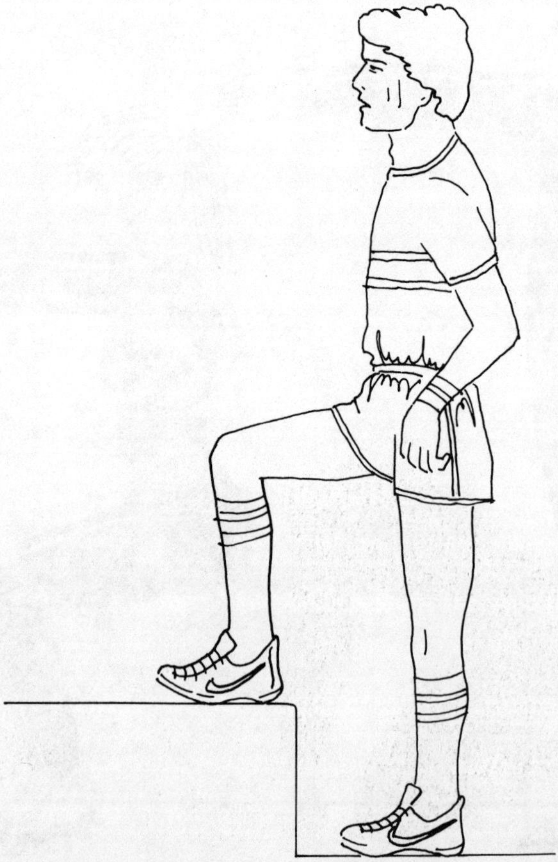

5. Sit-Ups: Have someone hold your feet or put your feet under a heavy couch or chair. *Be sure to bend your knees.* When doing sit-ups, tuck your chin onto your chest and roll up and back at a moderate pace. Clasp your hands behind your neck, elbows pointed ahead (pointing elbows straight out is more difficult). If you find that either of these positions is difficult at first, keep your arms at your side. Do five times.

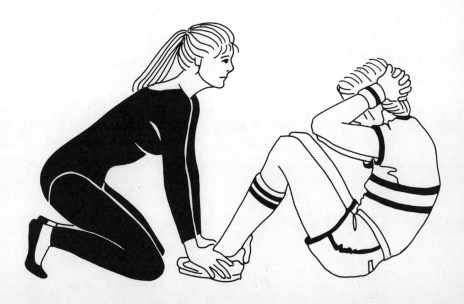

Level 4: Endurance

Now that you've devoted the month of January to getting in shape by improving your flexibility and strength, and by firming up your body, you should be ready to work on raising your capability to endure strenuous physical activity.

Don't be afraid. But don't be too enthusiastic, either. Take it a step at a time. Marathon runners, champion cyclists, and long-distance swimmers weren't born at those levels. Even though your goal is not a marathon or a medal, you have to start sometime. Start small, then build to bigger things.

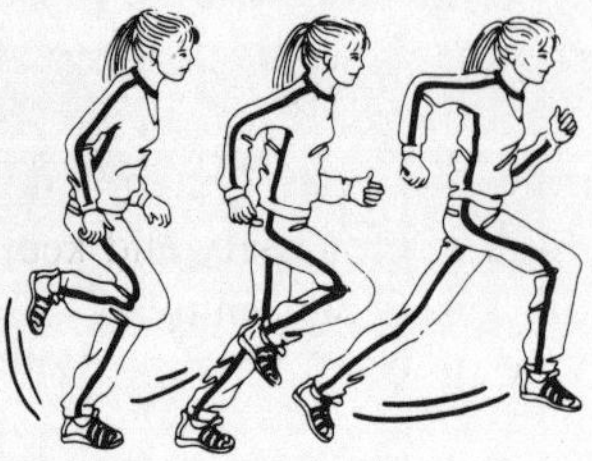

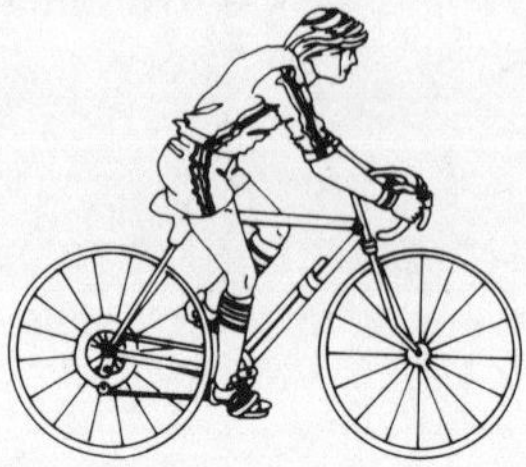

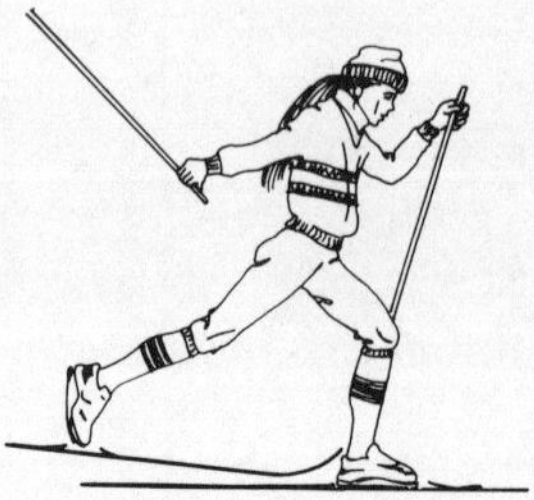

Here are the add-on flexibility exercises:

1. Groin Muscle Stretch: From a standing position with your feet three to four feet apart, slowly bend the right knee, and, while still facing forward, lean out toward the bent knee and hold the leaning position for five to eight counts. Repeat the groin muscle stretch four times with each leg.

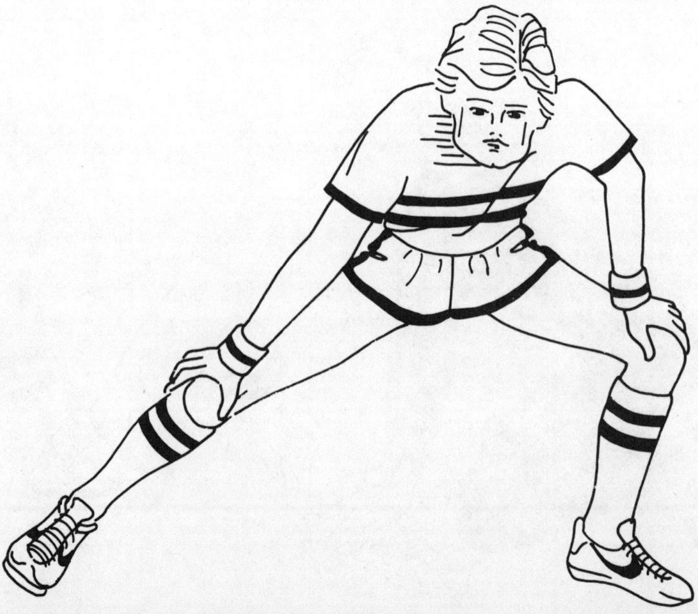

As you do every day, go through your 10 flexibility exercises. Then add the five new ones below, one a day, from January 30 through February 3. Only after you have done these 15 warmup exercises should you undertake your endurance activity.

Which activity? That is up to you. You can walk (as briskly as you can), cycle (at home or on the road), or swim (preferably in a pool). Cross-country (nordic) skiing is also very good , but not downhill (alpine) skiing.

If you are adding jogging, take a few precautions. When you walk, at any one moment you have a foot on the ground or floor. Not so for jogging. You bounce from one foot to the other. Be sure you strike the ground with your heel and roll onto your toes. Don't land on your toes or on the balls of your feet. Landing flat-footed is OK, but not as good as the heel strike. Wear the best shoes you can buy. If you run on a track, run in one direction one time, the other direction the next time, in order to prevent stress on the side you lean into.

Whichever activity you do, keep it up for 10 minutes. And breathe deeply as you do. Stay at this 10-minute level for two weeks. Then go to 15 minutes of activity and keep that level for another two weeks. Then go to 20 minutes—your goal is 30 minutes.

Cool down by doing one each of the first flexibility exercises, slowly.

2. Sprinter's Stretch: Squat down and place your hands on the floor in front of your body. Put your right knee up toward your chest and between your elbows. Extend your left leg behind your body. Hold for five to eight counts and just let your body weight stretch your leg muscles from this sprinter's position. Switch legs and repeat three times with each leg. *Do not bounce.*

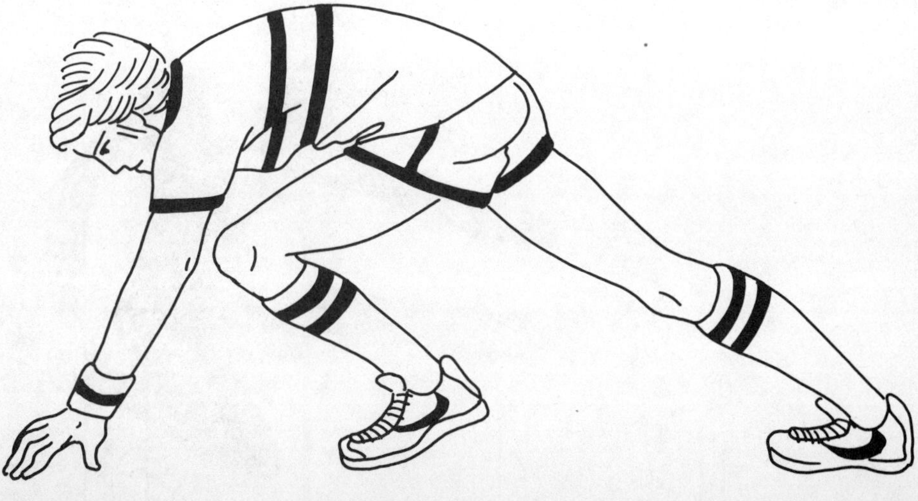

3. Hurdler's Stretch: Assume the sitting position illustrated with one foot tucked up next to your buttocks and the other extended in front of you. First, reach out toward the toes of your extended leg and hold for five to eight counts. This allows for the stretching of the muscles on the front side of the thigh of your bent leg. Repeat this procedure one more time on the same leg. Then switch leg positions and start from the beginning. *Do not bounce.*

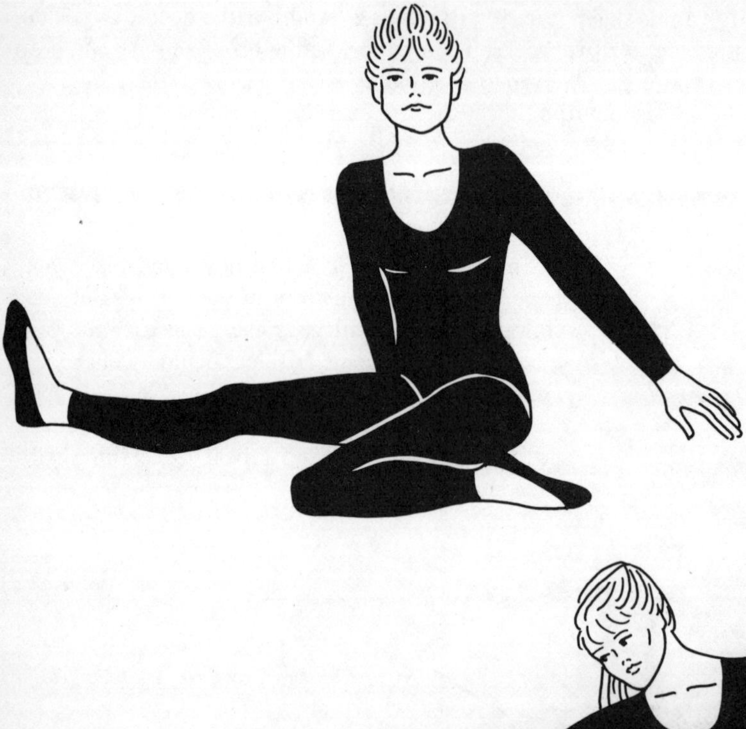

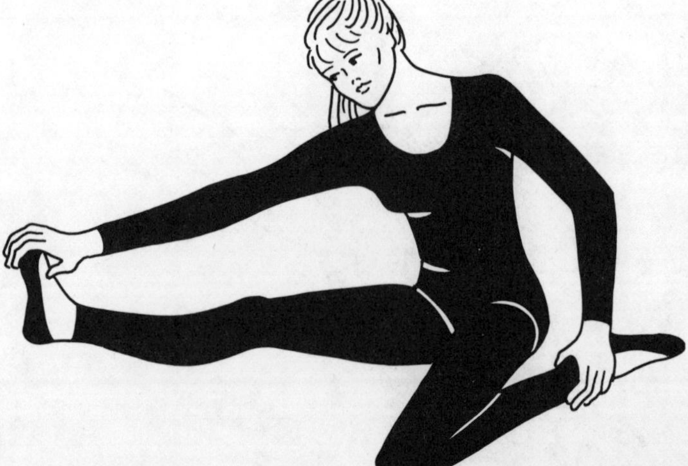

4. Double Calf Stretch: Stand at arm's length from the wall. Reach out and touch the wall with your hands. Slowly lean forward, keeping your heels on the floor and your body straight. Hold this position for 5 to 8 seconds and repeat three times. Be sure to keep your feet firmly planted on the floor.

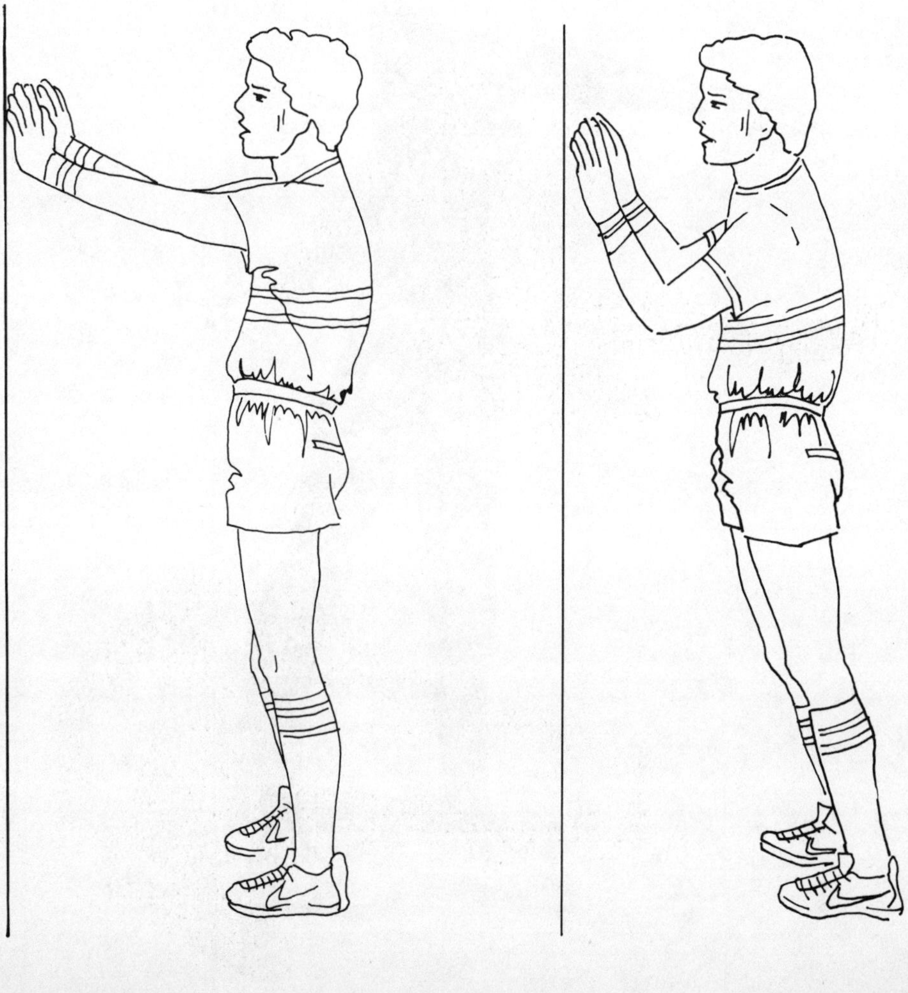

5. Crawl Stroke: Bending slightly forward at the waist, rotate your arms, alternating in large circles from your shoulder joints. This motion is similar to the crawl stroke in swimming. This may be done while you are in a walking or in a standing position. Do the stroke forward for 30 seconds then backward for 30 seconds.

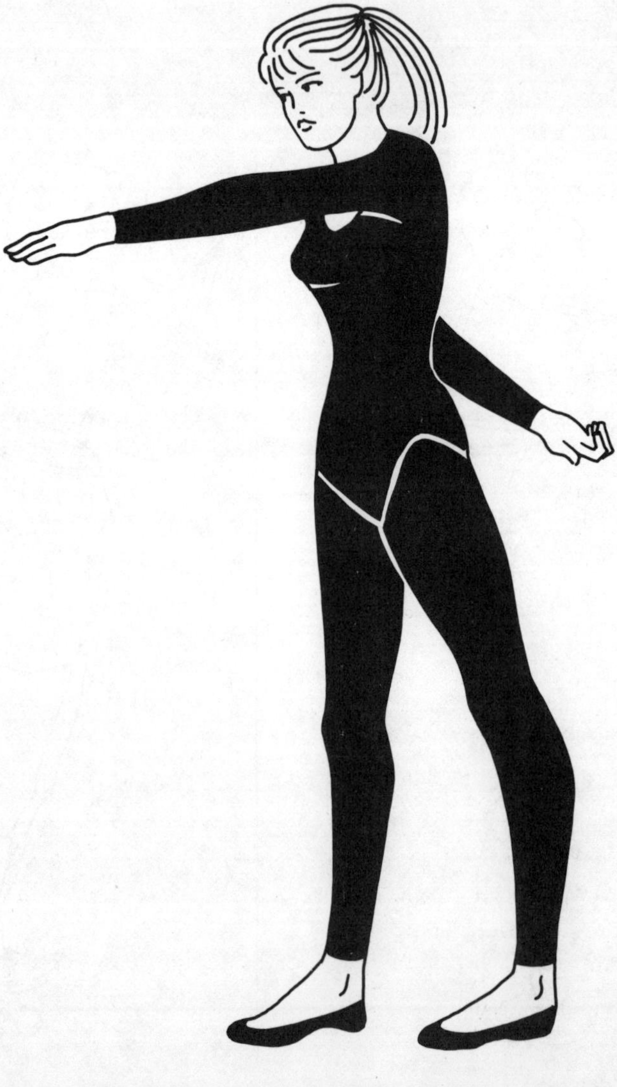

Staying on the Exercise Plan

It's April 1. By now you should be in top form. Congratulations. In three months you have built up your strength and endurance so that you can briskly walk, jog, cycle, or swim for 30 continuous minutes. And you do 35 different exercises, some every day, some every other day.

If you started your *Dieter's Almanac* Exercise Plan on New Year's Day, you should now have achieved this goal.

Here is your exercise plan for the rest of the year, one that will help you to stay in shape:

- Do the 10 basic flexibility exercises every day.
- Add the extra 5 flexibility exercises on the days you walk, jog, cycle, swim, or ski cross-country.
- Alternate endurance-building days with strength-building days.

At some time, you probably have had (and will have) some aching muscles. Treat these aches and pains as signals from your body. The muscles that are "talking" to you are the ones that were the most out of condition. Be gentle, but concentrate most on them.

Don't let your aches persuade you to stop exercising. Don't let them make you come to the conclusion that exercise is boring.

Don't falter! The aches will leave, and there are ways to cut boredom in exercising. One of the best ways to stay interested is to have an exercising buddy (preferably a sexually attractive one).

If you exercise indoors, play your favorite kind of music or even switch on a TV program. Out-of-doors you can use a radio or tape headset, not only to entertain you but also to keep your ears warm.

You'll soon find that exercising is great for relieving nervous tension, especially the kind you get from your work. You'll find yourself a more relaxed person at work and away.

Just as you have learned to exercise, so you must learn to relax. You must relax. Your muscles have to be worked, but they also have to be given the opportunity to rest and recover.

If you are the kind of person who needs to schedule relaxation on your calendar, do so. A little every day and a lot on the weekend. If you need a special technique in order to relax, learn it. Techniques that work well include meditation, yoga, tai chi, biofeedback, and autogenic training. So does sex. Stay away from alcohol and drugs.

A hot bath or a sauna are also good ways to relax. And either one will help banish whatever muscle aches remain.

To get to your goals requires determination and costs some time and pain. But it is worth it. When you are there, you'll be fit and strong and lean. And you'll feel better about your body.

THE DIETER'S ALMANAC

JANUARY

1st WEEK	If one of your New Year's resolutions is to exercise more, this week offers advice on how to start.
2nd WEEK	Resolved to quit smoking? You can do it without gaining weight. Just follow Mark Twain's advice.
3rd WEEK	A hot toddy takes the chill away, but it leaves fat behind. A guide to warming but low-cal drinks.
4th WEEK	Homebound and snowbound, especially with your family, promotes nibbling and laziness. Six rules for survival.

FEBRUARY

1st WEEK	The new school semester is a good time to look at how your children learn to eat—and overeat.
2nd WEEK	On Valentine's Day, examine your love for food and how it affects your human relationships.
3rd WEEK	George Washington is a good model for dieters. Tall, thin, and athletic, he ate sparingly.
4th WEEK	Lent provides an opportunity for thoughtful insights into your cultural and emotional dependencies on food.

MARCH

1st WEEK	If you come on to your diet like a March lion, you may suffer from "dieter's headache." These are ways to prevent it.
2nd WEEK	Going vegetarian is a good way to lose weight, if you know what foods to eat in proper combination.
3rd WEEK	St. Patrick's Day can play tricks on your diet. A guide to foods and drinks of the day.
4th WEEK	Here it is spring, and with it may come a reawakening of the urge to get in shape. How to start safely.
5th WEEK	Pick a partner to help you stay on your diet and conquer your compulsions about eating.

APRIL

1st WEEK	April Fool's Day! C'mon, sucker, buy the promises of the diet hucksters to melt fat away instantly!
2nd WEEK	Thomas Jefferson, whose birthday is this week, ate modestly until he traveled to France as Secretary of State.
3rd WEEK	Passover and Easter have the same religious root, the same emphasis on feasting, and the same emotional links to food.
4th WEEK	This is a good time to look around for a summer camp devoted to dieting, for yourself or your children.

MAY

1st WEEK	More people start dieting now than at any other time of the year. How to pick a diet for yourself.
2nd WEEK	D is for daily diet. Make sure it gives you all the nutrients you need to stay healthy as you lose weight.
3rd WEEK	I is for integrity. Every diet should have it. The original, prudent New York City diet did, and it is still a good one to adopt.
4th WEEK	E is for exercise. It helps take weight off and firms you up. A guide to calories and exercises.
5th WEEK	T is for training yourself to develop good new eating and exercising habits. It's called behavior modification.

JUNE

1st WEEK	The key to successful outdoor sports is to pick the one that best fits your lifestyle and preferences.
2nd WEEK	Fresh fruit in great variety is at the market. Some of it is loaded with calories. A guide to the best.
3rd WEEK	For Father's Day, a dozen rules for wives who want to help their husbands lose weight.
4th WEEK	The Great American Diet, compliments of the U.S. government, is the one to go on in preparation for the Fourth of July.

JULY

1st WEEK	Founding father Ben Franklin ate a near-vegetarian diet when he was a young man. He lived to be 84.
2nd WEEK	If you are planning a long auto trip, here are guidelines to keep you from racking up pounds along with the miles.
3rd WEEK	To prevent getting heat cramps during summer exercise, get enough water and salt.
4th WEEK	Camping and boating don't have to be pig-outs. Plan ahead and shop accordingly.
5th WEEK	Summer coolers and thirst quenchers taste great but are often laden with calories. Here's a guide.

AUGUST

1st WEEK	This is a good season to get lots of fiber into your diet. Fiber helps you lose weight and keep your health.
2nd WEEK	Salads are wonderful now, but not always the best dishes for dieting. How to pick ingredients.
3rd WEEK	Summer's here, so now is the time to plan your winter sports activities. Join health clubs carefully.
4th WEEK	Prepare for indoor exercising by buying a suitable indoor machine. A consumer's guide.

SEPTEMBER

1st WEEK	Labor Day (pun intended) is a good time to look at the nutritional needs of pregnancy, which is no time to diet.
2nd WEEK	As kids go back to school, make sure the lunches they take or buy are nutritious and light on calories.
3rd WEEK	The Jewish High Holiday of Yom Kippur offers a look at what fasting does to the body. It's not beneficial.
4th WEEK	Do you really need a hot breakfast? Do you need any breakfast? Well, it depends on your body's needs.

OCTOBER

1st WEEK	World Series fever comes from eating too much while watching the game at the ball park and on TV.
2nd WEEK	In honor of Columbus Day, take this quiz and discover anew how smart a dieter you are.
3rd WEEK	Humans are the only animals who eat when they're not hungry. That ability served a purpose in the past, not now.
4th WEEK	Skating and skiing are wonderful sports. To enjoy them this winter, start preparing your body now.
5th WEEK	Halloween is a diet disaster that teaches children that the treat is the trick. How to combat the evil.

NOVEMBER

1st WEEK	Here's how to keep slim as you go about your morning rituals. The tips come from the famous LaCosta Spa.
2nd WEEK	Appetite is still largely a scientific mystery. Here's what little we do know about it.
3rd WEEK	For Thanksgiving, let's go back to the modest fish-and-game dinner the Pilgrims had at Plymouth Plantation.
4th WEEK	Walking is the world's favorite exercise, and it's a good one to boot. Start a walking program today.

DECEMBER

1st WEEK	You don't have to stop jogging in the winter. You can even jog on snow. Here's how to do it, and how to care for your feet.
2nd WEEK	This is the dangerous season for serious dieters. The Hazardous Cs are everywhere. A dozen rules for surviving.
3rd WEEK	Here are the best Christmas gifts for a dieter. None of them costs money. Drop a hint to your spouse and friends.
4th WEEK	Most dieters can't go it alone; they need a group. A guide to the major diet organizations.

January—Week 1

If one of your New Year's resolutions is to exercise more, and you are hung up on how to start, here is some sound advice. It comes from Dr. Charles O. Dotson and Dr. D. Laine Santa Maria, two physical education experts at the University of Maryland.

Both stressed moderation. "I wouldn't recommend jogging to begin with. I would recommend walking," Dr. Dotson said. "During the first couple of weeks of your reconditioning plan, walk about a mile a day, three to five times a week."

The idea of walking, he explains, is "to give the joints, the tendons, a chance to recondition themselves." While muscles are very adaptable and can take more than moderate stress, your joints and tendons cannot. "They are the ones that seem to go first, and so we develop muscle soreness, joint pains, and even some complications."

At first it probably will take about 20 minutes to walk a mile. After a few weeks of regular walking, increase your pace until you are able to walk a mile in 15 minutes. Then walk briskly. Step up to a jog-and-walk, and finally try jogging the entire mile. Eventually you will do the mile in 8 minutes.

You don't have to stick with jogging. It is just a good way to get your body into shape. After you have reached that plateau of conditioning, you can swim, play tennis or handball, ride a bicycle, or do any form of vigorous exercise you prefer.

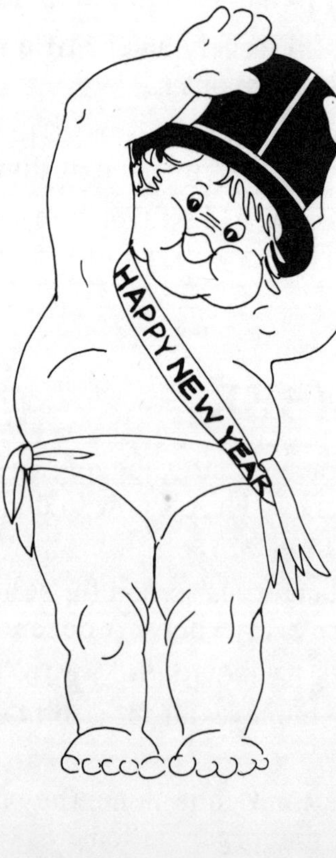

Dr. Dotson believes very strongly that "the exercise should be of the aerobic type, which means that you have to use oxygen while you are exercising." To use oxygen while you are exercising requires that you work for a minimum of 8 minutes.

In terms of calories, you burn off 5 calories per quart of oxygen you consume every minute. So the more vigorous the exercise, the more oxygen your muscles require, and the more calories you burn.

Dr. Dotson estimates that on a monthly basis you can, by exercising regularly, "burn in the neighborhood of 3,000 to 3,500 calories, which is equivalent to about one pound of fat." At this rate, by December you can lose a dozen pounds.

Conceding that this is a rather slow loss of fat, he stresses that if you diet *at the same time*, exercise can help you lose a significant number of pounds in a year.

Dr. Santa Maria offers a quick formula to determine if you are exercising strenuously enough. Check your heartbeat after you stop exercising. Count the number of beats for 15 seconds and multiply by four. That gives you the number of beats per minute.

Compare your exercise rate against what your maximum rate should be. If you are male, you get the maximum by subtracting your age from 220. Thus, if you are 40 years old, your maximum heart rate is 180. Your proper exercise rate should be 65 percent of that, or 117.

Women have a naturally higher heart rate. So subtract your age from 230 if you are female. If you're a 40-year-old woman, that would be 190 times 65 percent, or 124.

Here's another guide: "If your heart rate doesn't return to normal within 15 minutes you have exercised too much. If, after you have stopped exercising, you count your pulse and it is still 100 after 15 minutes, you have done too much exercise," cautions Dr. Dotson. Normal heart rates are 65 to 80 beats per minute.

Your breathing rate, too, should return to normal after 15 minutes. Normal is 12 to 15 breaths a minute.

Dr. Santa Maria cautions those too eager to get started in January: "I think the tendency for most people is to try to do too much in the beginning when they are starting on an exercise program." As a result, they get sore and discouraged and decide that exercise is not for them. So start slowly.

But start. Turn to the chapter on the *Dieter's Almanac* Exercise Plan and learn about the three-month program, which you start *now*. Follow the plan, and by April 1 your body will be flexible, firm, strong, and capable of a half hour of strenuous activity.

January—Week 2

Next to going on a diet, the most popular New Year's resolution is probably to quit smoking cigarettes. Such resolutions often go up in smoke when the tobacco addict is worried that many pounds of fat will accumulate after giving up the habit.

That you must gain weight after you quit smoking is part of the folklore of America. You've heard it before and you've seen friends and relatives who, once they quit, developed paunches and second chins. So, why risk it?

Also, you know about lung cancer and emphysema from smoking. But what about heart disease and diabetes from overweight? Which is the greater risk?

The health-risk question is easier to answer. Medical studies show that the rate of serious illness and death lessens among people who stop smoking—even if they do gain some weight.

The weight-gain question has been answered: "Not everyone who stops smoking gains weight. Of those who do gain, many gain only modest amounts." This answer appeared in the *Archives of Environmental Health*. It was part of a report based on a study of 501 telephone installers and repairmen by Dr. George W. Comstock of Johns Hopkins University and Dr. Richard W. Stone of the medical department of American Telephone and Telegraph Co.

They compared the weight of the men when they were first examined and five years later. They also noted whether the men were smokers.

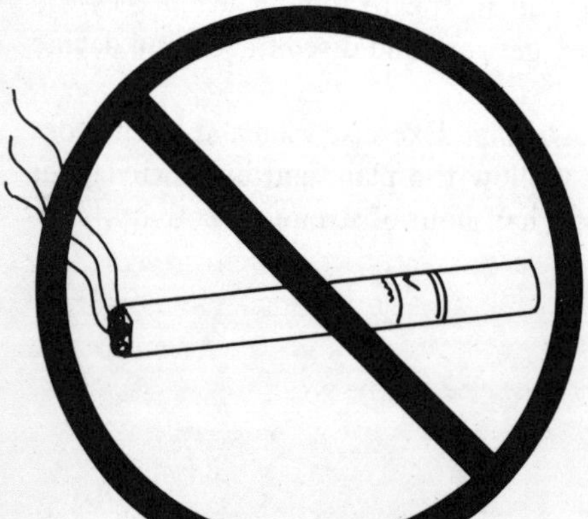

One general finding was that men who smoked cigarettes at the first examination weighed less on the average than those who did not smoke. The difference was between 6 and 11 pounds. Their other significant finding was that among those who quit smoking during the five years, seven out of eight gained weight. Their average weight gain was 4 pounds.

A team of Boston researchers who studied 870 healthy men who came every five years to the Veterans Administration hospital for checkups found that age was a stronger factor in putting on weight than was quitting smoking. A quarter of the smoke quitters either lost weight or remained the same. But, whether they smoked or not, men younger than 50 tended to gain weight, while men older than 50 tended to lose weight with the years.

Other studies, at Columbia University in New York, indicated that individuals who quit smoking on their own "were at least two to three times more successful than were people in other studies who went for professional help," according to Dr. Stanley Schachter in *Psychology Today*. And, the more times they tried to quit, the more successful they were liable to be, and the longer it had been since they last smoked.

Incidentally, the same was true of dieters, Dr. Schachter found. That is, people who dieted and lost weight on their own were far more successful in keeping it off than people who sought help in dieting from doctors or groups.

Concluded Dr. Schachter: "It may be that success rates with multiple attempts are greater than with single attempts, with or without the benefit of professional help." In both groups—smokers and dieters—the success rate of do-it-yourselfers was about two-thirds, or better than 60 percent. That compares with about 20 to 30 percent in diet groups.

If you resolve to quit smoking, prepare yourself. You are going to have to replace those cigarettes with something. Ready yourself by stockpiling both sugarless gum and hard candies, as well as celery and carrot sticks.

The most successful dieters and smoke quitters follow this advice from Mark Twain: "Habit is habit, and not to be flung out the window by any man, but coaxed down the stairs a step at a time."

You have to recognize that smoking is a habit, like nibbling, and that it has a strong hold on you. Particularly, it has a hold on you because of the mouth involvement. If you cannot smoke, you'll want to use your mouth anyway. Prepare for that. Find something else to do with your mouth, especially during the first days and weeks of quitting. Use those no-cal candies and gum and the chewy vegetables. Also drink diet soda pop and plain ice water. Whenever you feel that you need a drag, turn to one of these substitutes instead.

Also, your smoking is a ritual. You take the cigarette pack; you pick out, or pound out, a cigarette. You place it in your mouth. You light it with lighter or match, put that away, and take your first inhalation. Well, you have to replace that ritual behavior with something else—like getting up, going to the water fountain or the coffeepot, and filling up and taking a drink.

Exercise, too, is a good alternative activity to smoking. Turn to the *Dieter's Almanac* Exercise Plan and see how to get physically active *now*.

You'll slip. But you'll succeed if you keep trying. And you won't have to gain a pound. Or if you do, you'll be able to lose that pound in no time.

You can do it. Just coax your habit down the stairs.

January—Week 3

Nothing cures the chill of winter so well as a hot beverage. But on a diet, you have to carefully select the hot stuff you drink, lest it contribute unwanted calories.

For instance, what sounds so wonderful on a cuttingly cold winter night as a steaming cup of hot chocolate or hot cocoa? If you make it at home, from scratch with whole milk, that steaming cup of brown brew will cost you about 240 calories. The premixed kind, which you may get on the ski slopes, is about 120 calories a cup. And the diet versions made with skim milk powder are about 70. Marshmallows are 25 calories each.

If you prefer warmth from hot alcoholic drinks, you may tend toward a hot toddy. With the heat you also get a total of 200 calories per glass, derived from the sugar and the brandy or rum; the slice of lemon, nutmeg, and boiling water are "free." Or how about hot buttered rum? Its 190 calories are mainly derived from the square of butter and 2 ounces of rum. Or grog, with its 225 calories coming from the teaspoon of sugar and 3 ounces of rum.

Here are some other hot alcoholic drinks and their caloric prices by the glassful:

Drink	Calories
Brandy blazer	140
Glogg	305
Hot brandy flip	313
Hot buttered wine	175
Nightcap	315
Tom & Jerry	405

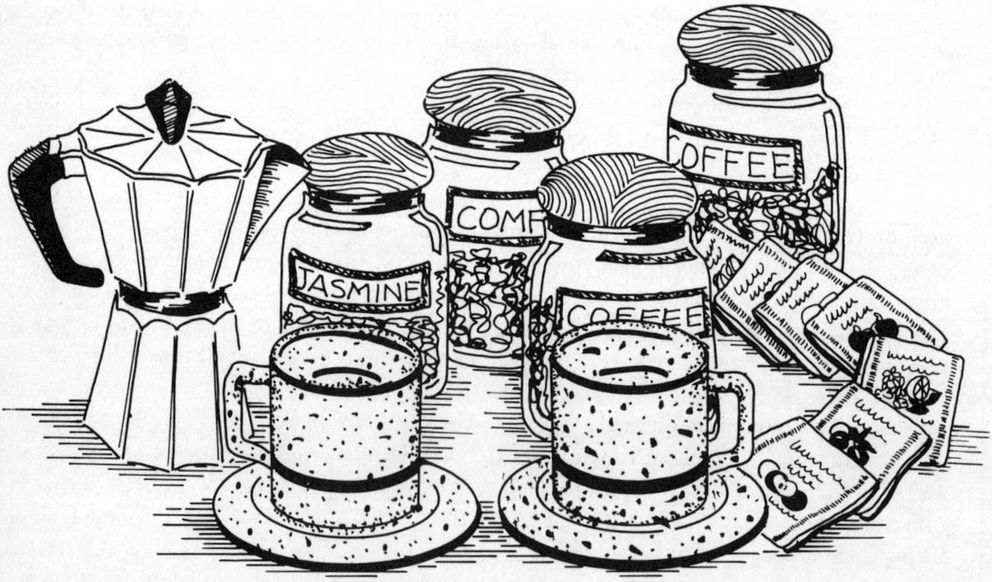

There are also versions of hot coffee that contain alcohol to heat you up. The "cheapest" is a cafe royal for about 40 calories a cup. Next best is orange-and-lemon-flavored cafe brulot (made famous by Brennan's of New Orleans) at 120 calories a cup. Irish coffee, which is very popular in some cities, costs you 155 calories a cup, thanks to its sugar, whisky, and whipped cream.

If you drink plain black coffee you can escape with about 35 calories. But adding sugar costs you an additional 15 calories per teaspoonful. Add half-and-half, and you get 20 calories per tablespoon more.

The fancier cups they serve in chic coffeehouses can cost you plenty. Here is how.

Espresso is a Continental coffee drink made in a special machine that forces steam and boiling water through finely ground Italian roast coffee. By itself, espresso yields few calories. But it is too strong to drink straight. Most people have to sweeten it to taste. If you use saccharine, you'll sweeten it without adding calories. But add sugar, and you pay 15 calories per teaspoonful.

Capuccino is espresso served with steamed frothy milk and cinnamon. Add another 50 calories. Chocalaccino is a variation in which capuccino is topped with whipped cream (10 calories per tablespoon of the frothy stuff) and shaved semisweet chocolate (at 145 calories per ounce). So drinking a cup of the delightful brew could give you 250 calories.

Cafe Dante has oranges and cinnamon for flavor, along with hot chocolate and whipped cream, for a total of 160 calories per cup. Plain homemade cocoa (with milk) is 245 calories a cup.

Cafe au lait and Viennese coffee are simply equal parts of coffee and milk, to which sugar and whipped cream are usually added, for 110 calories a cup. Some of the instant mixes sold in the supermarket are better because they contain nonfat dry milk, so you only get 50 calories per cup.

You can warm up with plenty of flavor and far fewer calories by turning to tea. There are fragrant teas made of flowers, such as camomile and jasmine. There are scented teas such as Earl Grey, which are combinations of Indian and Ceylonese to which bergamot oil has been added. And there are those wonderful commercial blends of spices with oranges or lemon or cinnamon. Any of these teas can be sipped by the cupful, giving no calories if you drink them straight or add just a bit of saccharine to the pot.

You don't even need a blend. Pour a basic tea such as Darjeeling or Russian black into a cup containing a cinnamon stick, and you have a delightful drink to warm you, free of calories. You can perform the same magic by pouring American coffee into a cup with a cinnamon stick, or with a dash of ground cinnamon, or both.

Another way to warm up, one that *uses* calories rather than packs them away, is exercise. Turn to the *Dieter's Almanac* Exercise Plan to find out how to start. If you have already started, you'll be doing strengthening exercises this week.

January—Week 4

The depths of winter can be disastrous for your weight, especially if you live in a northern clime. And winter is at its ultimate worst if you are snowbound.

Dr. Henry A. Jordan ought to know. He lives on a farm outside Philadelphia, which often gets heavy snows in January. He, his wife, and six children are immobilized at least once each winter. Dr. Jordan, a psychiatrist on the medical staff at the University of Pennsylvania, works with groups of overweight people at his Institute for Behavioral Education.

"This is a bad time for dieters. They are bored. They are confined. Their physical activities are limited. They can't even get out to see me, or to attend Weight Watchers or some other dieters' group.

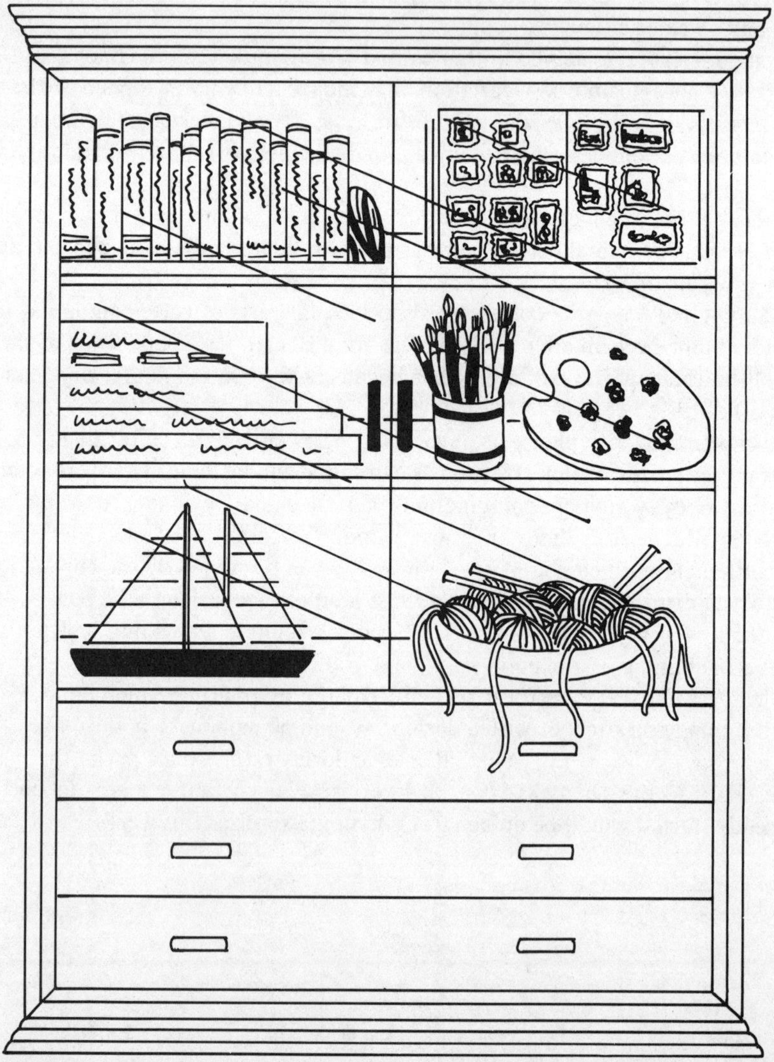

"But there is a positive light. If you can't drive to the supermarket, you can't load up on foods you shouldn't be eating. If you can get there by walking, the exercise will do you good and you'll buy only the essentials that you can carry home."

Nevertheless, shopping shouldn't be the limit of your physical activity. Dr. Jordan advises that you follow an indoor winter exercise schedule to temporarily replace your jogging, racquetball, tennis, swimming, or other favorite sport. He suggests calisthenics, rope skipping, running in place or on a treadmill, or an exercise cycle. Also the stairs, if you live in an apartment building or in a home not built on one level. (Or follow the *Dieter's Almanac* Exercise Plan.)

Keep your hands busy as much as possible, he says. "In our home, we have a hobby cabinet reserved for shut-in days. It contains jigsaw puzzles, games, and needlework. I have an office at home, which offers plenty of opportunity to keep me busy."

He suggests four ways to combat the doldrums, those feelings of blues and boredom that drive so many homebound dieters to the cookie jar.

1. *Keep in contact with the outside world.* Television is one way. Also use the phone to talk to friends and relatives. *Caution:* One of the most dangerous devices for dieters is the phone with the 15-foot cord that allows you to wander about and open refrigerator and cabinet doors as you chat.

2. *Keep in mind that this season is only temporary.* Spring will come, and you will be able to get back to normal activities in a couple of months.

3. *Plan a winter holiday.* Depending on your budget, it can be a trip to the sun or a weekend at a nearby lodge or spa. The planning will provide a light at the end of the tunnel and will give you a realistic goal: looking good at poolside.

4. *Enjoy the snow.* As you wait out the winter, romp in the snow with your kids. Build a snowman. Throw snowballs. Take a walk in the white; the fresh air will do you good and so will the physical activity, even if it is only for 5 or 10 minutes.

Some additional half-dozen rules for shut-in behavior come in Dr. Jordan's and my book, *The Doctor's Calories-Plus Diet* (New American Library, N.Y., 1982).

1. *Don't dawdle in the kitchen.* It is the food combat zone, with booby traps everywhere—in every cabinet, on every shelf, in the refrigerator. Every time you find yourself there, question why. The kitchen should not be the family room or library; it should serve no other purpose than meal preparation and consumption.

2. *Don't eat to kill time.* If you are bored, get involved in some activity other than working your jaws.

3. *Avoid ordering-in.* It just activates party behavior. Food brought into the house is considered special and OK to gorge on, even if it is not on your diet. Also, the portions are big, and the calories are usually intense.

4. *Don't put snacks in open dishes.* Nuts, pretzels, candy, and other finger food broadcast cues to be eaten. The more that food is visible, the more it tempts you to eat it.

5. *Take small portions.* Take less than you can eat, and do *not* take seconds. Eat slowly to make the smaller portions last longer than they otherwise would. If you feel compelled to ask for, or get, seconds, stop, wait 5 minutes, drink some noncaloric beverage, and take some deep breaths until the compulsion passes.

6. *Let someone else clean up the leftovers.* Keep them in small containers, so if you are tempted later, there won't be much there to eat.

Finally, Dr. Jordan advises: "Remember, these are unusual days. It's OK if you don't lose weight. A more realistic goal now is to maintain. Think of it this way: if you don't gain, you are way ahead. Congratulate yourself."

February—Week 1

With many youngsters starting a new school semester, now is a good time to take a look at how children learn an important behavior—eating. Let's especially look at how they learn to overeat, which is the basic cause of overweight. This examination should lend some insights into your own eating problems as well as help prevent them in your children.

The more that scientists reconstruct the natural history of obesity, the more certain they are that overweight adults were condemned to their problem by overzealous mothers who overfed them as babies.

A Michigan State University study suggests that the obese infant is usually the mother's first-born or is otherwise a new experience for her, such as her first premature infant or the first offspring she intended to breast feed.

In any case, the mother is oversensitive about the baby's fussiness and she finds that the nipple quiets baby. Soon she puts the real or plastic bottle nipple in baby's mouth whenever he (or she) cries. Secretly, say the doctors, she lacks confidence in her mothering and is reassuring herself: "See how much I love my baby, I'm busy feeding him all the time."

This constant feeding does something else for baby besides making him overweight. It also stunts the growth of his self-control. To quote the MSU doctors, the overfed baby is "left with an inability to distinguish his hunger drive from other drives and to

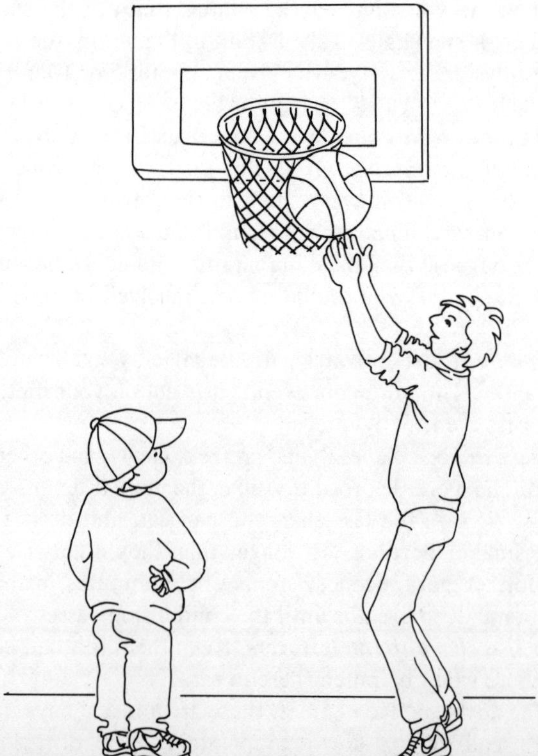

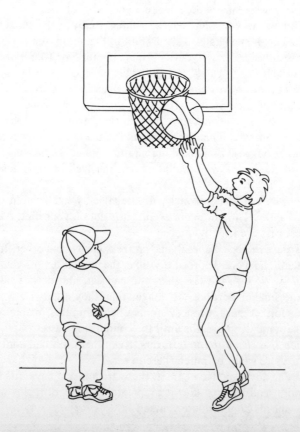

ascertain when he is satiated." These babies start lives in which they never know when they have eaten enough.

Such overfeeding of babies is "undisciplined, costly, and potentially harmful" in the opinion of three Johns Hopkins University experts, based on their study of the feeding of 109 Maryland youngsters at ages 2, 7, and 18 months. Dr. David M. Paige, Dr. Juan M. Baertl, and Dietitian Nancy H. Palmer found that at each of these ages the babies were being fed 30 to 40 percent more calories than government recommendations.

At 2 and 7 months, the youngsters were being fed far too much protein. The younger infants were unnecessarily being given cereals and strained meats, and the older infants were being given too much table meat and eggs as well.

The study showed that once baby can take solids, Mommy stuffs cookies, cakes, and other desserts into his eager mouth, as well as adding sugar to cereals and other dishes. Ten to fourteen percent of unnecessary calories come from sweets. This, said the Baltimore team, "results in overfeeding of most nutrients contributing to a potential problem of obesity and degenerative disease later in life."

If you see yourself as a new parent in these data, here is what to do about it. First, talk to your pediatrician and with a dietitian. Get a diet plan tailored to your baby. Most doctors simply pass on to new mothers a printed diet plan supplied free by baby food companies. (And you know what they are selling.)

Also, deal with baby's fussiness by means other than the bottle. Try holding, cooing, stroking, and hugging. The worst thing you can do is teach your child to eat when he or she feels nervous or upset. That is the kind of behavior that overweight adults have before they learn to get their strokes from folks and not from food.

If your children are taught proper, unemotional attitudes toward food early in their lives, they can go through life slim. By the time they are in school, or even in college, it is tougher for them to change. Still, it can be done. Some advice for college students comes from Dr. Frank Konishi, professor of nutrition at Southern Illinois University, Carbondale.

He notes that college men have more of an eating problem than coeds. "Many of the fellows established an eating pattern in high school, especially if they were involved in sports. They come to college, do not take up athletics and are not as physically active, but still eat as though they were. The result is they keep putting on pounds."

More pertinent is his observation that students usually put on pounds from between-meal eating. Beer drinking is one such consumption. Another is snacking. Continues Konishi: "Students keep food in their rooms and nibble when they study, when they are lonely, when they are anxious over tests or romances. This is because they were taught to put something into their mouths whenever they hurt or felt uncomfortable. When they were children, their mothers gave them pacifiers and their doctors gave them suckers."

College students should take a nutrition course to learn about the functions of food in the body; they already know about its emotional uses.

If your children are younger, you can teach such nutrition principles earlier in their lives. And you can teach them how to stay slim by setting the example. After all, *you* are their role model in life. The future physique of your baby is up to you now. The hand that rocks the cradle and holds the milk rules the scales.

That knowledge, too, will help you control your own eating habits and curb food abuses. (If you are on the *Dieter's Almanac* Exercise Plan, you start endurance exercises this week.)

February—Week 2

Valentine's Day is a good time to examine your loves—for another person and for food.

In her book, *Too Much Is Not Enough* (McGraw-Hill, 1981), self-admitted compulsive eater Sandra Edwards states, "Food is a lousy lover. Seductively silent, it tantalized, teased, and drew me toward it. Food tempted my sight and smell, my touch and taste. . . . Food was easier to get along with than a lover. With food, gratification was immediate. Gratifying sexual experiences required someone else, they took time and they were risky. . . . And food was illicit. It was a backstreet affair. . . . Food was the excuse I used to avoid knowing a lover. If the truth be told, I used food to keep any possible lover from knowing me. Especially my body. And I had infinitely more choices of food than of lovers."

Psychotherapist Mildred Klingman of New York City observes that "fat people very often ruin sex for themselves by refusing to allow themselves to enjoy it. They worry about the effect of fat on performance, and they are preoccupied with what their own body looks like—the flab and the sags and the cellulite, the lumps and bumps and stretch marks, and the just plain fat. They are all wrapped up in themselves. Sexuality, the ability to let go, is never given a chance."

In *The Secret Lives of Fat People* (Houghton Mifflin, 1981), she notes that the new openness about sex "is twice as inhibiting for fat people . . . their sex lives do not bear scrutiny under the new standards of ecstatic multiorgasms and no hangups."

In *Fat Is a Feminist Issue* (Berkley, 1978), England's Susie Orbach tells the story of Mary: "Her eating binges occurred almost uniformly when she was in any kind of potentially sexual situation. She would gorge away before going to a party, for instance, and convince herself that she was too big to be considered sexual." Fat served as her protection against sexuality. It prevented sexual advances that she could not handle.

For Mary, food was love: "She turns to eating in the search for love, comfort, warmth and support—for that indefinable something that seems never to be there."

Orbach thus reminds us that being fed is one of the first expressions of love that we

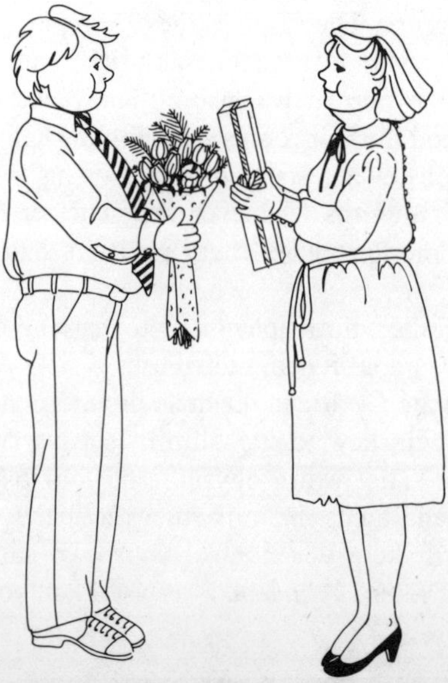

perceive. When you feel deprived or deserted, you eat. This happens often when you are alone, especially at night. That is why you raid the fridge in the lonely dark hours.

Now for the positive side of sex and weight.

Sex Therapist Barbara E. Bess found that not all fat people shun sex. In fact, their large appetites for food are often matched by large sexual appetites. But the prejudices of society are against them. "Obese persons want to be loved and sexually involved, but their bodies make them feel totally unlovable and sexually unappealing," Bess told the 1982 convention of the American Society of Bariatric Physicians. "As a consequence of the anxieties regarding their bodies, these obese may be inhibited in initiating sexual encounters. . . . Though sexual desires persist, they limit their sexual opportunities."

So, on this Valentine's Day, you as a dieter should dedicate yourself to two propositions. One is not to let excess pounds interfere with your love, lusts, and linkings. The other is to do something about removing those excess pounds that keep getting in the way.

Dr. Morton Walker and Joan Walker, both of the New Way of Life Weight Control Center at Stamford, Connecticut, have derived ways for couples to lose weight together, based on their experiences with clients. The key is communication.

In *Help Your Mate Lose Weight* (Jove, 1980), they explain: "You are the mirror of your mate. You are his or her determinant in weight-loss failure. You can build self-esteem or destroy it."

The most important way for your mate to help you is to be your friend. The Walkers offer a three-ingredient recipe for achieving friendship with mates.

1. *Trust.* Exchange your feelings openly, knowing that neither of you will use those feelings to hurt the other.

2. *Reveal.* Don't be afraid to expose what is inside your heart and mind.

3. *Communicate.* If your mate knows how you feel, he or she will be able "to visualize the temptations and addictive powers of certain foods. . . . Those special anxieties that so frequently sweep through any fat person will be made very real."

When your mate achieves this, say the Walkers, he or she will be able to see how the world looks to you, the dieter, how you can be "a compulsive consumer and possessor of an appetite that never sleeps." Not until this is accomplished can you and your mate deal on an intellectual level with problems of eating.

According to the Walkers: "Reducing accumulated pounds is a long and lonely business under ordinary circumstances. But the communication of mates on a feeling level can break down the loneliness." They point out that people who have been together for years have to start anew and reprogram their old attitudes. Couples often withhold true feelings for fear of hurting each other, invoking anger, or being rejected. This can be reversed by self-disclosure.

The Walkers' self-disclosure technique is for man and woman to keep a daily diary in which each records feelings during occurrences all day. Then, at the end of the day, in the privacy of the bedroom, they exchange diaries. After each reads what the other has written, they talk about it. This brings forth the emotional intimacy that can be matched by sexual intimacy.

That brings us back to sex. If your mate enjoys you in bed, and lets you know it, you'll want to look nice, to be slimmer. "The bedmate's emotions, expressed verbally or nonverbally, can motivate an individual to alter his or her appearance by losing weight, firming the body through exercise, practicing new sex techniques—anything to restore sex appeal for mutual joy in bed," advise the Walkers.

So heed this Valentine's Day advice for all lovers: Tell your love, and show it.

February—Week 3

Patriotism isn't the only reason to examine George Washington's diet as his birthday approaches. A better reason is that the Father of Our Country, like many fathers, is a good role model for those who are younger.

At age 26, Colonel George Washington was described by a fellow officer as "straight as an Indian, measuring 6 feet 2 inches in his stockings," weighing 175 pounds. He was very muscular, broad shouldered, and had long arms and legs. Tall for his times, his weight would be in the middle of normal on today's height-weight chart.

As a young Virginia farmer, Washington was less concerned with eating than with rotating crops, fertilizing the soil, and raising livestock on the 8,000-acre Mount Vernon farm he'd inherited from his half-brother, Lawrence. While George Washington participated in the gentlemanly pursuit of foxes on horseback, he also was rugged enough to break colts and wrestle other men.

Unlike Benjamin Franklin, Washington wrote nothing about his eating habits or the meals his servants or his wife prepared. The few accounts of his diet are scattered in the writings of persons who broke bread with him at one time or another. From these, we are able to construct his spare diet, one that could well serve dieters today.

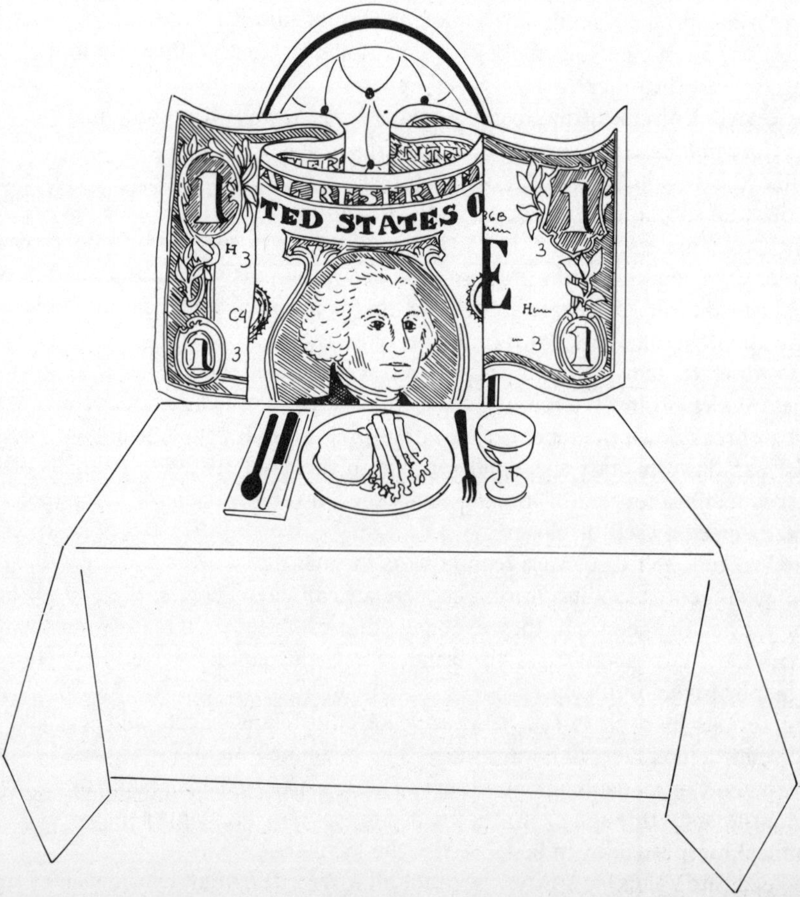

His meal schedule was breakfast at 8 A.M. (in the summer, it was 7 A.M.), dinner at 3 P.M., and supper early in the evening.

A 1794 breakfast served by Martha to George and a guest, Henry Wansey, consisted of dry toast, untoasted bread and butter, sliced tongue, and coffee and tea. If you assume moderate portions, this calculates to a total of 388 calories.

A 1779 dinner at West Point offered ham, "shoulder of bacon," roast beef, beans, and greens. Washington usually washed down his dinner either with cider or beer. (Water wasn't to be trusted then.) Again, assuming moderate portions of ham and beans, plus a glass of beer, he ate a total of 531 calories for dinner.

Washington's supper was really more of a snack, consisting of toast or some "well-baked bread" and tea. That would be only 218 calories. And so to bed, perhaps with a glass of Madeira (84 calories), his favorite wine.

This would give Washington a day's total of 1,221 calories, which is about what most dieters eat today. With it came 65 grams protein, 40 grams carbohydrate, and 45 grams fat. When you consider his physical activities on the farm, plus the fact that to get anywhere he had to walk or ride horseback, you can see why he stayed slim and muscular.

As far as historical consultants can tell, the same moderation was not practiced by Washington's neighbors in Virginia or by visitors to his dinner table in New York when he was President. For instance, a typical plantation breakfast of the time included muffins, waffles, biscuits with hung beef, bacon, tongue, fruit and cream, cucumbers, radishes, tea, and coffee. Any way you figure it, that's upward of 900 calories, just for breakfast.

A state dinner served by President and Mrs. Washington on August 27, 1789, attended and reported by William MacLay, included soup, fish, roasted and boiled meats, gammon (cured or smoked ham), fowls, and so on. Dessert featured apple pies, puddings, ice cream, and jellies. Also, watermelon, musk melon, apples, peaches, and nuts. Bread, wine, coffee, and tea were also served.

That he ate sparingly and stayed slim no doubt was an important factor in Washington's living to be 67, an advanced age in his time and place. The average life expectancy during his youth in Virginia was only 28. And had Washington not been bled to death by doctors treating him for sore throat, he might have lived much longer.

All in all, George Washington should be first in the hearts of dieters such as yourself. His life should serve to remind you that eating moderately and exercising strenuously will help keep your figure slim and your years abundant.

There is one hitch. Times were harder and food was scarcer two centuries ago than they are now. As we approach the twenty-first century, food is more abundant than ever in our society, and there is increasing urgency in messages that beckon us to eat, eat, eat. In this respect it is much more difficult for you than it was for Washington to eat sparingly.

On the other hand, portliness was a sign of high status in Washington's day, while slimness is "in" now. So he probably felt many pressures to gorge and grow fat. Yet he resisted them, just as he resisted the British in the Revolutionary War. As he fought the Redcoats and won, so he fought the gluttons and won.

The message on his birthday is that you can win too. Take command of your will and beat back the tired old forces that occupy your appetite and food habits. Then you can say, as he did, "It is well."

February—Week 4

Lent is a good time to look at the reasons behind your cultural and emotional links to food—which foods you eat and how and when you eat them.

The late E. O. James, when a professor at the University of London, defined in the most succinct way how Christ, his Apostles, and other founders of the early church organized and established food uses and taboos, in relation to religious observances.

In an article titled "Cultural and Religious Taboos Related to Food," James wrote: "Wednesdays and Fridays were observed as the weekly fast days, and the season of Lent, of varied durations, as the preparation for Easter, in the opening centuries of the new era." Lent, according to James, was intended as a preparation for the Easter festival, and over the centuries it has ranged from 40 hours to 40 days. First it was voluntary, then obligatory. It stemmed from Plato's concept of the body as the prison-house of the soul. "Hence, the need to bring it into subjection by strenuous abstinence and mortification," wrote James. This led to the Christian custom of receiving Holy Communion as the first food of the day.

Of course, few people can fast 40 hours, let alone 40 days, if by fast you mean complete abstinence from food.Today, Lent means limiting the intake of food on certain days. The Mardi Gras in New Orleans and similar festivals mark the preparation for Lent. They are ways of gorging, packing in calories to serve later in Lenten food cutback. In France there also used to be Refreshment Sunday, a carnival in mid-Lent, a gorging break.

The feast of Easter is closely linked with the feasts of Passover, one of which was Christ's Last Supper. The Christian feast is modeled after the predecessor Hebrew feasts, which in turn were based on pagan feasts of spring. (The word *Lent* comes from an old English word for spring.) Explained Professor James: "The deepest human emotions have always been aroused by and concentrated on fecundity and nutrition as the most vital concerns of the human race at all times and all ages."

Thus, Easter and Passover have their roots in ancient rites of spring that celebrated the resurrection of the earth after the long "death" of winter. The seed and the egg, the symbols of this resurrection, display humanity's hopes for fertile soil and fertile womb.

Likewise, Christmas and Chanukah, while unconnected religiously, are both Festivals of Light. They occur roughly at the annual time of greatest natural darkness, the winter solstice, when our spirits ebb. Both holidays are affirmations of the belief that the light of the sun will return and that earth and womb will again stir with fertility, and our spirits will rise. Both celebrations, too, are expressed by feasting.

From such cultural and religious bases spring your fundamental emotional ties to food, some of which have caused you to overeat and gain weight. In order to lose weight, and what is more important, to keep it off, you have to look into your heart and soul and understand these ties. You have to be aware of food's use as surcease of sorrow, balm, relief, and comfort when times are bad. And to recognize how food expresses joy, happiness, and celebration.

Your emotional link to food started, of course, at your birth. If your mother fed you every time you cried, you soon got the message, expressed in the Jewish idiom, "Eat, eat, you'll feel better." This is exactly the feeling behind your nervous appetite when things go wrong.

Home alone at night? Go to the refrigerator and eat. ("You'll feel better.")

Frustrated by life's unexpected bad deals? Take a cookie from the jar. ("It's all right. You deserve a treat after what happened to you.")

Angry at your spouse, parent, boss, partner? Take a bite of that candy bar you have hidden away. ("I'll show him.")

Elated over your child's straight-*A* report card? Take the family out to dinner. ("We're proud of you. Let's celebrate at a nice restaurant.")

Look at the many occasions upon which you eat for reasons other than hunger, and you will see cultural-religious-social-emotional links in the chain of your eating habits and behavior.

Most of the time you are not even conscious of the connections. And that is the problem. You automatically reach for food or make arrangements to eat. You don't even think about food when you wander into the kitchen, stroll into a bakery or candy store, or find yourself wanting everything on the restaurant menu. You merely react. You have been programmed since birth to so respond—to use food and to rely on food in this way. And if you are a parent, you have unwittingly so programmed your children.

Food does more than smell good and taste good and feel good. It is a way of celebrating the resurrection of Jesus or the rescue of the Israelites from Egyptian tyranny or the bounty of the earth. Food gives you something to do when you are nervous or scared to death. It is a treat, a reward, a center of celebration. It is what we offer to a friend who has suffered a loss, what we use as an excuse to sit down and talk things out. It is part of our holiest services, a way of communing with God.

For all these reasons, in all these uses, food is an essential part of your thoughts and feelings. As long as you are unaware of this, you will continue to misuse food and will continue to be overweight or—having lost weight—you will put it back on again.

The reverse is also true. If you come to grips with your nonnutritional uses of food, you can trim them back to a minimum. You can start changing your habits and practices.

The most successful technique for this is called behavior modification. It is the technique of changing your habits by replacing them with other habits. For example, instead of raiding the refrigerator when you feel lonely, pick up the phone and call a relative or friend, even one in another city. Instead of shopping when you are hungry, shop after a meal and thus stem your impulse buying.

These are but two examples. We'll get further into behavior modification at various other places in the *Dieter's Almanac*. In the meantime, keep yourself conscious of your feelings when you eat. A good way to do this is keep a diary or use a calendar to mark down the time, how you feel, and what you are doing every time you eat something.

Start. Do it today. Then review your food diary a month from now. Will you be surprised!

March — Week 1

If you come to your diet like a March Lion, you may well suffer from headache. In fact, headache is one of the most common reasons people go off a diet. If that's your problem, perhaps understanding diet headaches can keep you on the road to slenderville.

Our source is "the Headache King," Dr. Seymour Diamond, who runs a headache clinic in Chicago and was president of the American Association for the Study of Headache, and of the National Migraine Foundation.

Dr. Diamond explains that dieters can suffer from three kinds of headache:

- Tension headache, caused by the nervousness of having to live without constantly nibbling
- Low blood sugar, which comes from limiting your intake of food, especially carbohydrates
- Caffeine withdrawal, caused by dropping chocolate, coffee, and such from your menu

The first of the three, tension headache, is the only psychological headache. It is caused purely by nerves, by your emotional reaction to the fear that you won't be able to satisfy your cravings for food. It is the reaction to your utter horror at the prospect of not being able to shovel food into your mouth whenever you feel like it (even when no one's looking).

The way to get over a tension headache brought on by dieting is to face the fact that even on a diet, you will get enough food to stay alive. (Fasting is something else.) Also, be confident that you will be able to conquer your bad nibbling habit and still not starve.

In tension headache, the muscles of your neck tighten. You can fight this headache by learning to take out the kinks and knots. Once in a while, drop your head so your chin is on your chest, then raise it all the way up. Next, rotate your head from shoulder to shoulder in exaggerated swings. Take a hot shower. A rubdown will help too.

Exercise is a good way to relieve tension headache. Regular exercise, which you perform long enough to make you sweat (20 to 30 minutes or more), can do wonders to loosen up your muscles, even neck and shoulder muscles that contract in a viselike grip that usually precipitates tension headache.

(This is another good reason to jump into the *Dieter's Almanac* Exercise Plan. If you started back in January, you're be up to 15 minutes of endurance exercises this week. If not, this is as good a time to start as any. It will help relieve your tensions. It will help get your body in shape for summer, with its abbreviated clothes, which comes right after this spring season.)

People who fast often suffer the worst kind of low-blood-sugar headache. Many diabetics know exactly how this feels—essentially, a vague pain in the head. It can even lead to migraine and precipitate one of those all-encompassing attacks of intense head pain, light sensitivity, nausea—the works.

You should never fast, except for religious reasons and then only occasionally. And don't skip meals. Instead, eat on a planned, regular routine. Follow an even schedule of meals and snacks.

Caffeine-withdrawal headache is also vague, somewhat like tension headache. If your diet calls for abstinence from chocolate, cola, coffee, and tea—rich sources of caffeine—don't go "cold turkey." Ease off gradually, recognizing that you are addicted and that unless you are careful, you will suffer the same drug withdrawal reactions as other addicts.

While aspirin is the most common treatment for headache, it does not mix well with dieting. That is true because much of the time, if you are on a strict diet, your stomach will be empty. Aspirin is an acid. Left alone in the stomach, it can cause heartburn, nausea, and worse. If you must take two aspirins, take them with a full glass of water and during a meal or snack.

Finally, advises Dr. Diamond, when you go on a diet, you are liable to start eating foods you were not eating before. If you are prone to headaches, these foods may contain substances that precipitate headache, such as sodium nitrite and tyramine. Look at the accompanying list of foods to avoid if you are trying to prevent headaches.

Diet for the Headache Patient*

Avoid:

Ripened cheeses (cheddar, Emmentaler, Gruyere, Stilton, Brie, and Camembert)

(Cheeses permissible: American, cottage, cream, and Velveeta)

Herring

Chocolate

Vinegar (except white vinegar)

Anything fermented, pickled, or marinated

Sour cream, yogurt

Nuts, peanut butter

Hot fresh breads, raised coffeecakes, and doughnuts

Pods of broad beans (lima, navy, and pea pods)

Any foods containing large amounts of monosodium glutamate (Chinese foods)

Onions

Canned figs

Citrus foods (no more than 1 orange per day)

Bananas (no more than ½ banana per day)

Pizza

Pork (no more than 2-3 times per week)

Excessive tea, coffee, cola beverages (no more than 4 cups per day)

Avocado

Fermented sausage (bologna, salami, pepperoni, summer sausage, and hot dogs)

Chicken livers

Avoid all alcoholic beverages, if possible. If you must drink, no more than two normal-size drinks.

Suggested drinks: haute sauterne, Riesling, Seagram's VO, Cutty Sark, vodka.

*From Seymour Diamond and Donald J. Dalessio, *The Practicing Physician's Approach to Headache* (Baltimore: Williams & Wilkins, 1978).

March — Week 2

Going on a vegetarian diet to lose weight is not so wild a notion. Some diets, such as Pritikin's, actually are semivegetarian diets. They exclude red meat and include some cheese, fish, and poultry.

You can understand the benefits of vegetarian cuisine when you consider that a 6-ounce sirloin steak packs 660 calories. That steak contains more fat than protein, and half of that fat is the saturated kind implicated in heart disease.

By contrast, broiled fish gives the same amount of protein without saturated fats and with only half the calories. Three cups of skim milk give the same amount of protein and no fat at all, for only 270 calories.

Plant-derived protein is often fat free and contains no cholesterol. You get thinner on a vegetarian diet than on a meat diet because you eat foods that are not highly packed with fatty calories. Also, vegetables and fruits are bulky and fill your stomach, holding off hunger. And they are rich in fiber, which moves digested food through your intestines and minimizes absorption.

This is not vegetarian propaganda. A team of Harvard University nutritionists, led by Dr. Johanna T. Dwyer, a few years ago studied 100 young vegetarians in the Boston area. "Weight loss is one of the most common medical findings," they reported in *Medical Opinion* magazine. Most of their subjects were at their lowest adult weights. Interestingly, men lost proportionately more weight than women did, perhaps because of the meat-and-potatoes male ethic.

While some of these vegetarians ascribed their weight loss to the philosophical or religious reasons that caused them to take up vegetarianism in the first place, Dr. Dwyer and her research team found that "the weight loss is not caused by some magical property of the vegetarian diet." The "Veggies" simply ate fewer calories than they did before.

But before you throw your meat into the garbage can and start stuffing lettuce leaves into your mouth, first study vegetarian diets in detail.

There are many versions, but a common ingredient in all vegetarian diets is an emphasis on foods derived from plants. Actually, "vegetarian" is misleading. While the diets include vegetables, they also include fruits, legumes, cereals, grains, nuts, and seeds. They exclude the flesh of four-legged animals such as cattle and hogs. Here are some vegetarian definitions:

- Vegans are strict, or pure, vegetarians who eat only plant foods.
- Lacto-vegetarians eat plant foods plus dairy products such as milk, cheese, yogurt, and ice cream.
- Lacto-ovo-vegetarians eat eggs as well as dairy products and plant foods.
- Semivegetarians eat fish and fowl once in a while, as well as eggs, dairy products, and plant foods.

If you are thinking about becoming a vegetarian, it's a good idea to check with your doctor before switching your diet. Because a vegetarian diet is a high-bulk diet, you should be sure you do not have an active gastrointestinal disorder such as peptic ulcer or ulcerative colitis.

Don't expect your doctor to be sympathetic; he probably doesn't understand vegetarian diets. But if he is knowledgeable about vegetarianism, he will caution you to take supplements of vitamin B-12. If you go on a vegan diet, you should also take supplements of vitamin D, calcium, riboflavin, and iron. The meat and dairy products you'll avoid are rich in these. Meat is the richest natural source of vitamin B-12.

Another problem with vegetarian diets is protein. The protein in animal foods—meat, milk, eggs—is complete. But the protein in plant foods is deficient. However, you can get complete protein by mixing legumes and nuts, and from soy protein and wheat.

To stay healthy and lose weight as a vegetarian, you have to know exactly what you are doing. Stay away from the dangerous diets, especially the Zen Macrobiotic and the rice diets. Do follow the diets of Seventh Day Adventists, who have this worked out. You can get lots of information from the SDA Dietetics Association., Box 75, Loma Linda, CA 92354. Another good source of information is the American Dietetic Association, 430 North Michigan Avenue, Chicago, IL 60611.

The best popular vegetarian books are: *Diet for a Small Planet* by Frances Moore Lappe (Ballantine, 1982), *Recipes for a Small Planet* by Ellen Buchman Ewald (Ballantine, 1973), and *It's Your World Vegetarian Cookbook* (Review & Herald Publishing Association, 1982). On all, be sure to get the *revised* edition, for all have been updated.

High-protein, meat-substitute entrees made from soybeans are available from:

Archer Daniels Midland Co., Box 1470, Decatur, IL 62525

A. E. Staley Mfg. Co., 2222 Kensington Court, Oak Brook, IL 60521

Cargill, Inc., Port Cargill, Savage, MN 55378

Central Soya Co., 1300 Ft. Wayne Bank Building, Ft. Wayne, IN 46802

Dawson Sales Co., Dawson, MN 56232

Far-Mar-Co., Inc., 960 North Halstead, Hutchinson, KA 67501

Loma Linda Foods, Riverside, CA 92505

Ralston-Purina, Checkerboard Square, St. Louis, MO 63188

Worthington Foods, Worthington, OH 43085

SEVEN DAYS' MENUS FOR 15% FAT LACTO-OVO VEGETARIAN DIET
1200 CALORIES

DAY 1

BREAKFAST	
Orange juice (frozen)	4 oz.
Banana, small	1 small
Rolled wheat	4 oz.
Raisins	2 tsp.
Milk, nonfat	8 oz.
LUNCH	
Baked potato, small	1 small
*Almond nut loaf with	4½ oz.
**Tomato gravy	¼ cup
Tossed salad:	
Tomatoes	1 lg.
Head lettuce	¼ head
Lemon-juice dressing	2 tbsp.
Whole wheat bread	1 sl.
SUPPER	
*Minestrone soup	1 cup
Celery sticks (5 in. long ¾ in. wide)	3
Whole wheat bread	1 sl.

TOTAL	
Calories	1202
Protein	52.
Fat	20.1
Carbohydrate	218.5

DAY 2

BREAKFAST	
Grapefruit	½
Fresh apple	1 med.
Roman Meal cereal	¾ cup
Dates, chopped	2
Milk, nonfat	8 oz.
LUNCH	
*Tostada Casserole	¾ cup
Mustard greens/lemon juice	¾ cup
Yellow squash	1 cup
Whole wheat bread	1 sl.
SUPPER	
*Soybeans Americana	1 cup
**Cornbread	1 piece 2 x 3¼"
Peaches, canned	2 halves
TOTAL	
Calories	1197
Protein	55.0
Fat	20.9
Carbohydrate	215.4

DAY 3

BREAKFAST	
Nectarine	2 med.
Oatmeal, cooked	½ cup
Raisins	2 tsp.
Milk, nonfat	8 oz.
Whole wheat bread	1 sl.
LUNCH	
*Cottage Cheese Croquettes	2
Beets, cooked	½ cup
Green beans, cooked	⅔ cup
Hot corn tortilla (6")	1
SUPPER	
*Syrian Bread Sandwich 1	
Seasoned garbanzos	⅓ cup
+Mediterranean Pocket Bread	1 pocket
Orange Juice	8 oz.
TOTAL	
Calories	1207
Protein	52
Fat	20.7
Carbohydrate	216.5

DAY 4

BREAKFAST	
Orange slices (2⅜ in. diam.)	1 sm.
Banana, small	1 sm.
Bran muffin	1
Milk, nonfat	8 oz.
Margarine	1 pat
LUNCH	
*Singapore Surprise	¾ c. sauce
with Brown rice	⅓ cup
Winter squash, baked	4 oz.
Whole wheat roll	1
Radishes (¾ in. by 1 in. diam.)	2
Cooked frozen okra	1 cup
SUPPER	
*Lentil Vegetable Stew	1 cup
Raw zucchini slices	½ cup
Whole wheat bread	1 sl.
TOTAL	
Calories	1190
Protein	57.2
Fat	19.2
Carbohydrate	216.7

DAY 5

BREAKFAST	
Orange juice (frozen)	4 oz
Pear, fresh Bartlett (2½ in. diam. 3½ high)	1
Bulgur wheat, cooked	4 oz.
Dates, chopped	2
Milk, nonfat	8 oz.
LUNCH	
*Danish Proteena Balls & Sauce	6 oz.
Brown rice	1 cup
Spinach, cooked	½ cup
Cauliflower, cooked	½ cup
SUPPER	
Onion soup diluted with water	1 cup
Carrot salad:	½ cup
Carrots, grated	3 oz.
Raisins	1 tbsp.
Pineapple chunks (H2O pack)	2 oz.
Corn, boiled	½ cup
Whole wheat bread	1 sl.

TOTAL	
Calories	1198
Protein	55.4
Fat	21.4
Carbohydrate	209.3

DAY 6

BREAKFAST	
Grapefruit	½
Berries, fresh	1 cup
Milk, nonfat	8 oz.
Cornmeal, cooked	1 cup
Almonds	2 tbsp.
LUNCH	
Cottage Cheese (3% fat)	½ cup
Tomato, sliced	1 (3½ oz.)
Green pepper rings (3 in. diam. ¼ in. thick)	4
Potato, baked	1 sm.
Brown Gravy Quik	¼ cup
Asparagus spears	½ cup
Whole wheat roll	1
SUPPER	
*Pink Creole Beans	1 cup
Celery sticks (5 in. long and ¾ in. wide)	3
Carrot sticks (1⅛ in. diam. 7½ in. long)	1
Whole wheat toast	1 sl.
Dried apricot halves	5
TOTAL	
Calories	1194
Protein	61.5
Fat	18
Carbohydrate	210.9

DAY 7

BREAKFAST	
Fresh pineapple, diced	1 cup
Papaya, with lime wedge	⅓ med.
Whole grain wheat cereal	⅔ cup
Fig, chopped	1 large
Milk, nonfat	8 oz.
LUNCH	
*Vitaburger on	1 lg. patty
Hamburger roll	1 roll
Cabbage salad	1 cup
Mayonnaise	1 tbsp.
Green beans	1 cup
Tomato, sliced	½ med.
Fresh apricots	6
SUPPER	
Tostadas:	
Corn tortillas	2 6 in.
Mashed pinto beans	¾ cup
Lettuce	½ cup
Diced tomato	1 sm.
Green pepper sticks	½ cup
TOTAL	
Calories	1205
Protein	58.7
Fat	18.3
Carbohydrate	219.4

+ Indicates recipes adapted from Century 21 Cookbook
*** Indicates unpublished recipes*
** Indicates recipes adapted from It's Your World Vegetarian Cookbook*

Courtesy Department of Nutrition
School of Health
Loma Linda University

ALMOND-NUT LOAF

1 cup almonds, sliced thin, toasted lightly
1⅓ cups Skallops, ground
1⅓ cups diced celery, sauteed lightly
2 tablespoons onion, minced finely
½ cup fine dry bread crumbs (whole wheat)
¾ cup evaporated milk
2 eggs
½ teaspoon sweet basil
1 tablespoon chicken-like seasoning

COMBINE all ingredients.
TURN into well-oiled loaf pan.
COVER with foil.
SET in pan of hot water.
BAKE AT 350 degrees F. until set; 55 min., uncover for a few minutes at end to brown.
8 servings.

TOMATO GRAVY

2 tablespoons diced onion
2 teaspoons oil
2 cups tomato juice
1 teaspoon salt
4 tablespoons flour
1 teaspoon celery salt

SAUTE onion in oil.

BLEND flour with ⅓ cup juice and seasonings.
COMBINE all ingredients and cook until thick, stirring constantly.

MINESTRONE SOUP

¼ cup garbanzos, dry
¼ cup red beans, dry
¼ cup pinto beans, dry
¼ cup navy beans, dry
¼ cup lima beans, dry
1 cup canned tomatoes
½ cup chopped onion
½ cup chopped celery
1 cup dry macaroni
1 teaspoons oil
1 teaspoon Accent
1 teaspoon salt
1 bay leaf
Minced parsley to garnish

BRING beans to boil in 4 cups of water.
TURN off heat and let stand 1 hour.
COOK until tender (about 1 hour more or pressure cook ½ hour).
ADD remaining ingredients and enough water to make thick soup.
SIMMER 30 to 40 minutes.
REMOVE bay leaf.

5 cups (1 cup per serving)

TOSTADA CASSEROLE

½ cup Vita-Burger
½ cup hot water
20 oz.can chile beans (Loma Linda or Worthington)
10¾ oz. can mushroom soup
4 crisp tortillas broken into pieces (not Fritos)
1 or 2 tomatoes, chopped
1½ cups lettuce, chopped

SOAK Vita-Burger in hot water 15 minutes.
COMBINE first five ingredients.
ALTERNATE layers of chips and Vita-Burger mixture in oiled casserole.
BAKE at 350 degrees F. for 20 minutes.
REMOVE from oven.
SERVE with lettuce and tomato as topping.

6 servings

BAKED SOYBEANS AMERICANA

6 cups cooked soybeans (3 cups dry soybeans / 12 cups water)
2 tablespoons molasses or a drop or two of maple flavoring
2 tablespoons brown sugar
juice of 1 lemon
2½ tsp. salt
1 can tomato soup or
1½ cups tomato puree
1 medium onion, whole

COOK soybeans:
ADD to boiling water; as soon as beans boil again, turn off heat. Let stand 1 hour.
SIMMER until nearly done. Add salt. Continue cooking until beans are soft. 1-2 hours depending on variety.
MIX all the ingredients except the onion.
PLACE in bean pot or baking dish. Put the whole onion in the center.
BAKE at 350 degrees F. 1 hour or longer, adding a little bean broth or tomato juice as needed to keep moist.

8 1-cup servings.

YEAST CORNBREAD

1 tablespoon yeast
1 tablespoon sugar
2½ cups warm water
1 tablespoon oil
2 cups cornmeal
2 cups wheat flour
½ cup wheat germ
1 tablespoon salt

DISSOLVE yeast and sugar in warm water.
ADD oil.
MIX together dry ingredients; then add yeast mixture to dry mixture all at once.
STIR only enough to moisten all ingredients. Lightly pat batter about ¾ inch thick into a prepared 9 x 13 in. baking pan. Let rise half again; then bake at 350 degrees F. for 45 minutes, or until done.

COTTAGE CHEESE CROQUETTES

¼ cup minced finely onion
1 tablespoon oil
3 eggs, beaten
1 teaspoon Spanish paprika

½ teaspoon sage
½ teaspoon thyme
2 tablespoons food yeast flakes
2 cups low-fat cottage cheese
1¼ cups fresh bread crumbs (whole grain)
¼ cup dry bread crumbs
½ teaspoon salt
1 can mushroom soup diluted with
⅓ can of water

SAUTE onion in the oil, add to eggs and seasonings.
ADD cottage cheese, crumbs, and salt. Blend.
FORM into patties. Fry in pan sprayed with no-calorie coating until golden brown on each side. Place in baking dish.
COVER with diluted mushroom soup.
BAKE 350 degrees F. for 20 to 30 minutes.

6 servings

SYRIAN BREAD SANDWICH (Eggless)

1 1-lb. can garbanzos (mashed with fork)
¼ tsp. garlic powder
¼ tsp. cumin
2 tsp. chopped parsley
1 tbsp. lemon juice
1 tsp. salt

MIX all together and refrigerate for at least one hour.

Shredded lettuce
Chopped cucumber
Chopped tomatoes
Chopped onion

PREPARE all vegetables and chill.

6 small loaves Syrian Bread

CUT bread across center and open. Half fill with first mixture and top with chopped vegetables.

6 servings

MEDITERRANEAN POCKET BREAD

2 pkgs. yeast
2 cups warm water
1 tbsp. brown sugar
2 cups unbleached flour

COMBINE in order given and beat until smooth, about three minutes.

⅓ cup oil
2 tsp. salt

ADD and mix well.

3 to 4 cups whole wheat flour

ADD to make a medium stiff dough.
KNEAD on a floured board until smooth, 5 to 10 minutes. Cover dough with bowl and let rest 30 minutes.
ROLL into a 16 inch log; cut into 16 pieces and shape into balls. Roll out into 5 inch circles.
PLACE on greased baking sheets.
LET RISE 30-45 minutes until puffy.
BAKE at 400 degrees F. on bottom rack about 10 minutes. Remove and cover while cooling.
CUT pocket in bread and fill with your favorite filling.

16 loaves

SINGAPORE SURPRISE

1½ cups rice (brown and wild rice mixed give excellent taste)
1⅓ cups boiling water
2 teaspoons oil
½ teaspoon turmeric for color (optional)
½ teaspoon salt
8 oz. frozen Luncheon Slices Smoked beef-like, torn into bite-size pieces or cut into small cubes
2 tbsp. oil
¼ cup flour
2 cups non-fat milk
1 8 oz. can water chestnuts, drained and sliced
1 10 ounce package frozen peas, cooked

COOK rice with water, oil, turmeric, and salt in covered, heavy kettle about 45 minutes.
SAUTE soyameat lightly in oil. Reserve small amount for garnish.
ADD flour to remaining soyameat in frying pan and stir well. Then add the milk, stirring constantly while it thickens.
FOLD in water chestnuts.
FOLD peas into rice.
SERVE sauce over rice.
GARNISH with sauted soyameat reserved for this.

8 servings

LENTIL-VEGETABLE STEW

1 cup lentils, uncooked
2½ cups water
1 medium potato, diced
1 medium carrot, sliced
1 cup celery, cut
½ cup onions, chopped
1 large bell pepper, diced
2½ cups water
6-oz. can tomato paste
½ cup Vita-Burger
2 teaspoons salt
½ teaspoon Savorex
½ teaspoon (scant) sweet basil

ADD water to lentils and bring to boil.
TURN off heat and let stand 30-45 minutes.
FINISH cooking until almost tender.
COOK vegetables in the 2½ cups water.
COMBINE all ingredients; simmer 20-30 minutes.

10 servings

DANISH PROTEENA BALLS

14 oz. can Proteena
1 cup tomato puree
2 eggs
½ teaspoon sage
2 tablespoons chopped parsley
½ teaspoon Savorex
1 medium onion, grated
1 tablespoon oil
½ medium green pepper, chopped
⅔ cup breakfast cereal flakes

MASH Proteena fine; add other ingredients.
ADD sufficient cereal to make medium soft ball.
FORM balls size of walnut; place in oiled 6 inch x 10 inch casserole.
BAKE at 350 degrees F. for 30 minutes.
BASTE with Danish Sauce before removing from oven.

DANISH SAUCE

1 tablespoon oil
1½ teaspoons Savorex
¼ cup evaporated milk
1 teaspoon cornstarch
½ cup water

ADD Savorex to oil and brown.
ADD milk; cook until it curdles. Add water in which the cornstarch has been blended.
COOK 5 minutes. This should be a thin sauce.

6 servings

PINK CREOLE BEANS

1 lb. dried pink beans
6 cups water
2 tablespoons oil
1 cup chopped celery
1 cup chopped onion
1 green pepper, chopped
1 cup tomato puree
2 cups canned tomatoes
2 tablespoons molasses
1 teaspoon Accent
2 tablespoons Soy Sauce
2 teaspoons salt
½ teaspoon sweet basil, rubbed

SORT over beans, wash.
ADD beans to boiling water.
BRING back to boil; cover, remove from heat and let stand 1 hour or overnight.
SIMMER until almost tender.
SAUTE vegetables in oil 1 minute at low heat.
ADD all ingredients to beans.
SIMMER 30-45 minutes until tender and thickened.

VITABURGERS*

1 cup Vitaburger*
1 cup hot water
3 tablespoons chopped onions
1 tablespoon flour
3 egg whites
sage

SOAK Vitaburger in hot water for 15 minutes.
ADD other ingredients and mix well.
COOK in prepared Teflon skillet.
**Granburger or TVP may be substituted.*

6 patties (using ⅓ cup for each)

March — Week 3

Sure and begorra, this is the time of St. Patrick's Day. And if you get swept up in the revelry—no matter what your background—you're apt to be loading up on calories.

I know that in Chicago everyone is proclaimed Irish on St. Patrick's Day. That gives one and all license to spend the day drinking and eating the fine brew and finer food. Woe to the dieter swept up by the throngs pouring out of office buildings at noon, making their way from bar to restaurant. Gone is the resolve, as back come the pounds.

You can blame it on the leprechauns if you want, but the truth is, 'tis you that breaks the diet and must suffer, not them. So here's a dieter's guide to St. Patrick's Day, so you can plan in advance what you should be eating.

You'll stop at one bar and swig down a good shot of fine Irish whisky. There you'll be given a kiss and a pin that says "Kiss Me, I'm Irish." On to another bar, where you have some Irish ale and a handful of pretzels to chomp on as you swap jokes.

Finally to the restaurant, after elbowing your way out of the bar. You have to wait for your reserved table to be cleared, so you start another ale, then sit down. You order some typical fare, such as Irish lamb stew or corned beef and cabbage, with boiled potatoes, rye bread and butter, salad with dressing. And you top it all off with Irish coffee. Was that a little elf with a clay pipe and green hat in the corner, winking as your caloric intake at lunch topped the thousand mark? Poof, and he's gone!

In many ways, St. Patrick's Day is very much the Halloween of spring. It is a time for people to let go, to masquerade, to be outrageous. It is as though all about you are mad, and madness is normalcy. How easy it is to be swept up in the orgy.

If you are a serious dieter, there is but one way to behave on this day: Stay home, or stay in your office. Brown-bag it. Resist all invitations and temptations to go along. Be firm but polite. (After you lose that extra weight, you may want to go along next year, or the year after.) Above all, don't trust yourself. Know that once you join the crowd, the social pressures you'll feel will force you to drink up and eat up. To help you keep your dieting resolve on St. Patrick's Day, here is a recap of the calories you would have consumed in the little vignette above. Hang on to your fork!

Food	Quantity	Calories	Fat	Protein	Carbohydrates
Corned beef	3 slices	183	10.2 g	21.5 g	—
Lamb stew	1 cup	220	6.0	6.0	40.0
Cabbage	3 cup	20	0.2	1.1	4.3
Potato	1	65	0.1	1.1	14.5
Bread, rye	2 slices	112	0.6	4.2	24.0
Butter	2 pats	72	8.2	—	—
Soda biscuits	2	240	6.0	6.0	40.0
Salad	small	25	—	—	—
Dressing	1 T	101	11.2	0.14	2.0
Ale	2 8-oz.	196	—	2.2	—
Irish whisky	1.5 oz.	119	—	—	—
Pretzels	2 oz.	235	3.0	6.0	46.0
Irish coffee	glass	220	4.0	—	12.0
Totals: Corned beef dinner:					1,349 calories
Irish stew dinner:					1,428 calories

March — Week 4

Spring is here, with summer not far behind. As the earth stirs with reawakening activity, you find yourself in one of two states:

- Physically fit and ready for outdoor sports and displaying yourself in shorts
- Out of shape, too embarrassed to wear shorts, and far from ready for outdoor sports

You're in great shape if you have kept up with the *Dieter's Almanac* Exercise Plan since the first of the year. If not, you can start now, and be in shape for the Fourth of July.

The worst way to proceed is to jump right in and try to make up for lost months in getting back in shape. This is often the tendency in people who are overweight, since many of them have the kind of personality that drives their behavior to compulsion. Such people typically dive in with abandon.

When they eat, they eat too much.

When they diet, they cut back too much on eating.

When they exercise, they push themselves beyond their limits.

When they are sedentary, they move barely a finger.

Sound familiar?

Before you rush off to jog 10 miles for the first time in six months, stop and read this. In exercise, as in everything you do, you need to be aware of what you are doing.

Exercise is a natural activity, of course, but it can hurt you. In order to prevent strains and other injuries, you have to observe four cautions.

1. *Warm up and stay warm.* Warm muscles are less likely to be injured. Start slowly with gentle, rhythmic exercises to ease tension. You will find that the more tense you are, the more warmup you will need. You should start perspiring before you really open up or get into play. And bundle up afterward to avoid chills.

2. *Train.* The best way to prevent strains and other injuries is to undergo long and conscientious training to strengthen proper muscles and tendons.

3. *Don't deny.* If you do hurt yourself, don't neglect it. Major injuries grow from minor injuries that are ignored. New injuries should be treated with ice packs; those that have been neglected for several days will respond to warm soaking.

4. *Reeducate.* Unused muscles weaken and become more susceptible to further injury. Thus a vicious cycle can occur. If you've been inactive for a week or so, exercise until the unused muscles have regained their former strength.

While I'm at it, I also want to caution you against static exercises. A report to the American Heart Association explained how these can be dangerous. Isometrics do not provoke the heart to beat faster, as it should, so it can keep pace with increased metabolic needs. Dynamic exercises such as swimming and running do make the heart beat faster.

According to Dr. Jere H. Mitchell of the University of Texas at Dallas, dynamic exercise causes large changes in muscle length, thus generating a demand for more oxygen; this in turn stimulates a call for more blood, which then makes the heart beat faster.

In static exercises, no such chain of events occurs. Dr. Mitchell reported that this is probably why "there are many stories of people who have died during heavy static exercise such as changing a tire or shoveling snow." He recommends that anyone who lifts weights or regularly practices other static exercise should add a dynamic exercise to the routine, so that the heart and arteries can keep pace.

Another report came from the Department of Transportation's study in Washington's tropical July heat and humidity. It compared bicyclists with motorists taking the same routes home at rush hour. The cyclists had higher incidences than motorists of fatigue, sore throat, and eye irritation. (But the motorists who rode in air-conditioned cars had more carbon monoxide in their blood.) Fortunately, said the researchers, the effects of heat and air pollution were temporary.

The same should apply to rush-hour urban joggers and anyone else dynamically exercising out-of-doors in summer in a city. So take those pollution and ozone warnings seriously.

This is not to discourage you from exercising if you've suddenly discovered that you are middle-aged, overweight, and underfit, and that the closest you have come to sports in the past 20 years is what you see on your TV screen. Runner and writer Hal Higdon, in *Fitness after Forty* (Anderson World Publications, 1977), quotes several authorities who made the point that the body does not have to deteriorate rapidly in middle age. Finding a fascinating parallel between physical fitness and voice, he echoes Wilma Osheim, a Chicago-area voice teacher: "If the voice is used properly, a person can sing in top form until the late 60's or even the early 70's." Properly cared for, a voice declines slowly. Decline in general athletic ability comes slowly too. In a cared-for body, tissues lose elasticity and nerves and muscles lose their precision coordination very slowly.

Most middle-aged flab and lethargy is not caused by a slowing of metabolism, but a slowing of oomph. In fact, Higdon quotes statistics showing that swimmers who keep in athletic condition after age 25 have an average fall-off in performance of only 0.8 percent a year. Similarly, 1,500-meter runners average a 3-second slowdown per year. Most of this slowdown comes from changes in the respiratory system.

One percent a year is a far cry from what most middle-agers experience. They probably decline more rapidly because they consider exercise a travail. "One of the greatest myths perpetrated on the American public over the last four decades has been the notion that exercise or physical activity is not fun," writes Higdon, who cites the triumph of students who come to gym with a doctor's excuse and snicker at classmates forced to exercise.

The best sport to start in middle age is the one you enjoy, because you'll stick to it more faithfully on a regular basis, not just every other weekend.

The point of all this is that exercise can do much to get and keep you in shape. But, as in any other activity, you have to know what you are doing. You have to know how to begin and when to stop. That's one of the differences between the "I tried it once" fatty and the "I do it daily" svelte.

March — Week 5

As a dieter in a world of eaters, you may sometimes feel like "E.T.": a lost soul on a strange planet. Take heart. You needn't be alone. And you don't have to join a diet club or group. You can ask a friend to help.

A diet partner, writes Dr. William Rader, "can be more helpful than an internist, psychiatrist, psychologist who has a dozen degrees." Rather than professional expertise, your partner "can offer you qualities that are essential to boost your self-esteem and change your relationship with food—namely, he can share his humanness, his genuine day-to-day concern, his closeness, his reason, his mutual problems, and his approachability." ("She" and "her" fit here too.)

In his book, *Dr. Rader's No-Diet Program for Permanent Weight Loss* (Warner Books, 1981), he offers six guidelines for choosing a diet partner:

1. Your partner should have a weight problem. You need a colleague who has a similar eating compulsion, and who has some of the same thoughts and feelings.

2. Your partner needs to be interested enough in losing weight to make a firm commitment to end compulsive overeating.

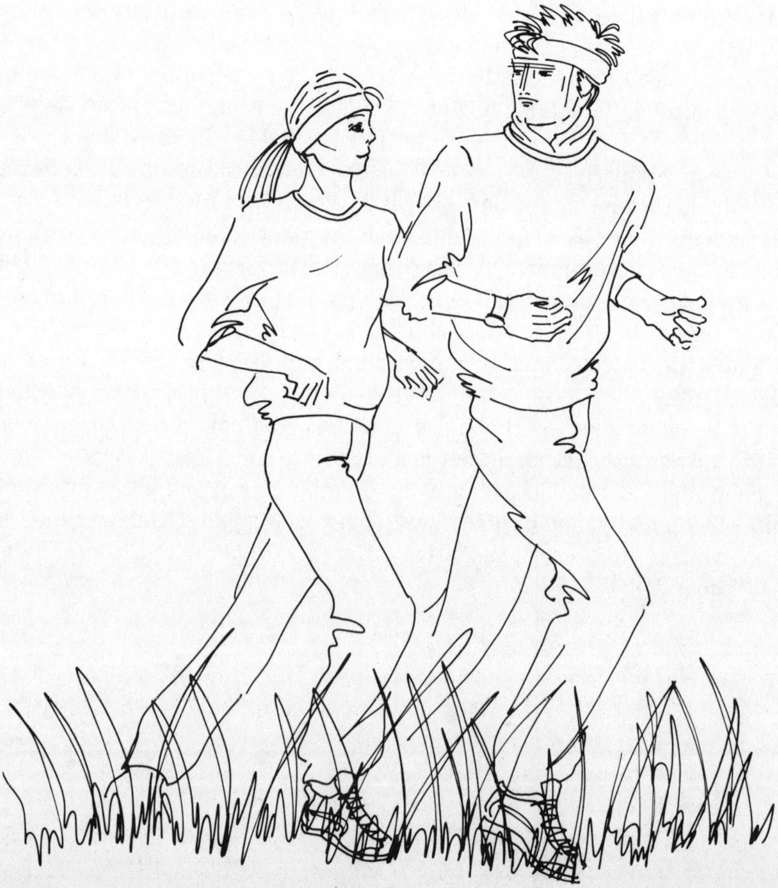

3. Your partner should not be someone you want to impress, but a person you feel close to and can be honest with.

4. Your partner should not be the kind of person who judges and criticizes you and offers unsolicited advice.

5. Your partner needs to be available for daily phone calls, twice-a-week meetings, and hastily convened get-togethers during periods of crisis.

6. Your partner should *not* be your spouse, parent, or other family member. Normal interpersonal conflicts and issues will get in the way.

Another diet doctor, Psychiatrist Kelly Brownell, of the University of Pennsylvania, doesn't completely agree. A spouse, relative, friend, or lover can be your diet partner, he feels, but it is not enough to want to help you. He or she has to know specifically what to do to help.

Dr. Brownell thinks a partner should not monitor *what* you eat so much as *how* you eat. He or she is part of your behavior modification program, the changing of your bad eating habits to good. Your partner is there to help you develop these habits.

Every slimming behavior you learn, you practice with your partner. He or she is there to compliment and encourage you when you're down, and to cheer you when you're up.

In *The Partnership Diet Program*, written with Irene Copeland (Rawson, Wade, 1980), Dr. Brownell explains that the person you are living with—mate, lover, roommate—may be the most logical partner. Or it can be a friend, neighbor, co-worker, even a relative. However, he advises, your "potential partner should be able to commit both time and emotional involvement to your effort." Don't choose someone who is too busy. If your partner is a dieter, all the better; but this is not essential.

Once you have a candidate, talk it over with him or her. It is especially important to explain how you want to be handled, that is, strictly or loosely. Then go over the partner's responsibilities. These include modeling good eating habits; keeping a daily food log; reinforcing your good behavior; praising your actions, not your weight loss; and conducting your important weekly weigh-in.

In his experience at his Philadelphia weight-loss clinic, Dr. Brownell found that understanding the dieter's problem is the most important thing a partner can do. Also, the partner must be a helper, not a manager. "The dieting process is like a bicycle built for two. When *both* people do the pedaling, you reach your destination faster and with a cooperative spirit that pleases everyone."

Dr. Rader says a good partner has to know how to listen effectively and respond constructively in twice-a-week meetings. That means not giving advice. "Rather, it entails helping your partner formulate, understand, and interpret his own thoughts and feelings and then decide for himself the most appropriate action he can take. You are there primarily as sounding boards for one another, to gently encourage and support each other as you sift through your respective experiences."

Mostly, a partner needs to encourage the friend to take responsibility for his or her own problems and actions, Dr. Rader advises. A partner best serves as a mirror for the dieter's words, letting him hear himself in a different way. Open with phrases such as, "What you seem to be saying, is . . ." That kind of reflection helps the dieter define feelings and become aware of subsequent actions.

And knowing how your feelings tie in with your compulsion to eat is the first big step toward changing such behavior and then losing weight. And, finally, keeping it off.

April — Week 1

When it comes to losing weight, even the smartest and the wisest, the best and the most brilliant can be fools.

Let April Fool's Day serve to remind us how easy a "mark" we are for the diet huckster, how gullible are the overweight, how fast we fall for the quick-weight-loss promise.

Yet the ads beckon. Witness:

CAN MAKE YOU SKINNY IN 45 DAYS . . . EVEN IF YOU CHEAT!!!
OR DOUBLE YOUR MONEY BACK

DISSOLVES STUBBORN BULGES AND WASHES AWAY YEARS OF BUILT-UP FAT

The promises persist:

- Shrink millions of fat cells in the first 24 hours.
- Melt off up to 10 pounds in 4 days.
- Continue to lose 30, 40, 50, up to 100 pounds or more if you need to.
- Thrill to fast weight loss without gnawing hunger pangs. *April Fool!*

Writing in the *Journal of the American Medical Association*, that organization's director of foods and nutrition, Dr. Philip L. White, notes "A final example of strange things people do in the interest of thinness is body-wrapping. Salons specializing in this practice have sprung up all over the country. The client is smeared with 'special creams' and then wrapped in plastic. So long as sweating is not too profuse or body temperature does not rise alarmingly, there probably is as little harm (to healthy people) as there is benefit from this practice. It does, however, serve to illustrate the lengths to which people will go to avoid proper dieting and exercise. Passive exercises, running a rolling pin over one's pudge, or submitting to little electrical shocks in sites of adiposity are other reducing methods that continue to attract many clients." *April Fool!*

Of late, these diets have been promoted for melting off fat: a diet that emphasizes lecithin, vinegar, kelp, and vitamin B-6; spirulina, a foul-smelling derivative of algae that grow in brackish subtropical ponds; and "starch blockers," a substance extracted from northern beans that is supposed to safely and effectively let you eat lots of starchy foods without absorbing any calories.

Over the years there has been an abundance of mail-order devices for removing fat without your having to give up gorging or to start sweating. There was a sky-blue inflatable plastic belt worn around your waist to sweat off inches in days. There were devices you plugged in that quietly stimulated your muscles and used up calories. And all manner of exotic mechanical devices for passively exercising your fat away. *April Fool!*

Then there are the pills and medicines.

In the 1920s you rubbed a cream on your skin. The cream harmlessly dissolved the fat below, said the ads, "leaving the figure slim and properly rounded, giving the lithe grace to the body every man and woman desires."

In the 1940s it was dried seaweed. Then came the spot-reducing vibrators and electric belts.

In the 1950s doctors pushed prescription drugs that cut back appetite. Some made local reputations and minor fortunes by prescribing these "pep" pills to the overweight. The pills, classified as amphetamines, worked for a while. Then the appetite came back. But the need for the pep pills remained. Countless patients couldn't get started in the morning without their pills. The medication was so effective that underground traffic began in what became known as "speed."

Amphetamines were brought under strict legal control and fell into disrepute. Finally, the U.S. Food and Drug Administration issued a regulation prohibiting doctors from prescribing amphetamines for weight-control purposes. The FDA did this because "amphetamines continue to be abused at a rate substantially higher than that for other drugs used in the treatment of obesity." *April Fool!*

Then the FDA announced that it was OK to sell another kind of drug over the counter, without a prescription, to stem appetite. The drug is sold under various trade names, such as Anorexin, Dexatrim, Prolamine, and Spantrol. Chemically, it is phenylpropanolamine, primarily used for years as a decongestant in such cold remedies as Contac. It curbs appetite as a result of its pep-pill-like side effect: stimulation of the central nervous system.

In reviewing reports on phenylpropanolamine, the *Medical Letter* found serious cases of illness and even death among heart patients who took it. It has also been implicated in kidney disease.

The FDA also approved the use of benzocaine, a local anesthetic sold for generations to fat patients by the patent-medicine men. Its gimmick is dulling your taste buds so that food loses its taste appeal. If you follow ads in magazines, you can tell that this deadening principle has been carried to an even more absurd level. One ad claimed you could "Spray your weight away!" The magic ingredient in the mouth spray is that old dental painkiller, benzocaine.

The bottom line on these drugs is this: They work, but weakly. Oh, they'll curb your appetite somewhat, and dull your taste sensations somewhat. But they won't work to help you lose weight over the long run. As the *Medical Letter* puts it, "There is no good evidence that phenylpropanolamine, oral benzocaine, or any other drug can help obese patients achieve long-term weight reduction. The only satisfactory treatment for obesity is a life-long change in patterns of food intake and physical activity."

To paraphrase Shakespeare, the secret to weight-loss lies not in the promises but in ourselves.

Still, the hucksters go on. The market is big; some 50 million Americans are overweight. That's a lot of dieters, especially if they can be persuaded to send in money for mail-order magic. How about half the total for only a buck apiece? That's a nice piece of change. *April Fool!*

You do have some recourses if you feel you've been taken. You can write to one or both of the following: Federal Trade Commission, Pennsylvania Avenue at Sixth Street, N.W., Washington, DC 20580; or Mail Fraud Division, U.S. Postal Service, 475 L'Enfant Plaza West, S.W., Washington, DC 20260.

And drop a line to your local Better Business Bureau, Chamber of Commerce, and newspaper as well.

(No fooling: If you've been on the *Dieter's Almanac* Exercise Plan since New Year's, you're at the top. You're able to do 30 minutes of running, swimming, walking, and other such endurance activities. Congratulations. Stay trim and in shape. If you haven't taken up the exercise program, start now, so you'll be in shape for summer.)

April — Week 2

Dieters could have no better hero than Thomas Jefferson, first Secretary of State, second Vice President, and third President of the United States. His birthday is April 13.

As author of the Declaration of Independence, founder of the University of Virginia, lawyer, architect, and inventor, his intellect was that of a creative genius. But his physique was also noteworthy. A contemporary said, "Mr. Jefferson was 6 feet 2 inches high, well-proportioned, and straight as a gun barrel. He was like a fine horse—he had no surplus flesh."

When he was young, his family called him "Tall Tom." One secret of his slimness was that he was always on the move. Many considered him the most industrious indi-

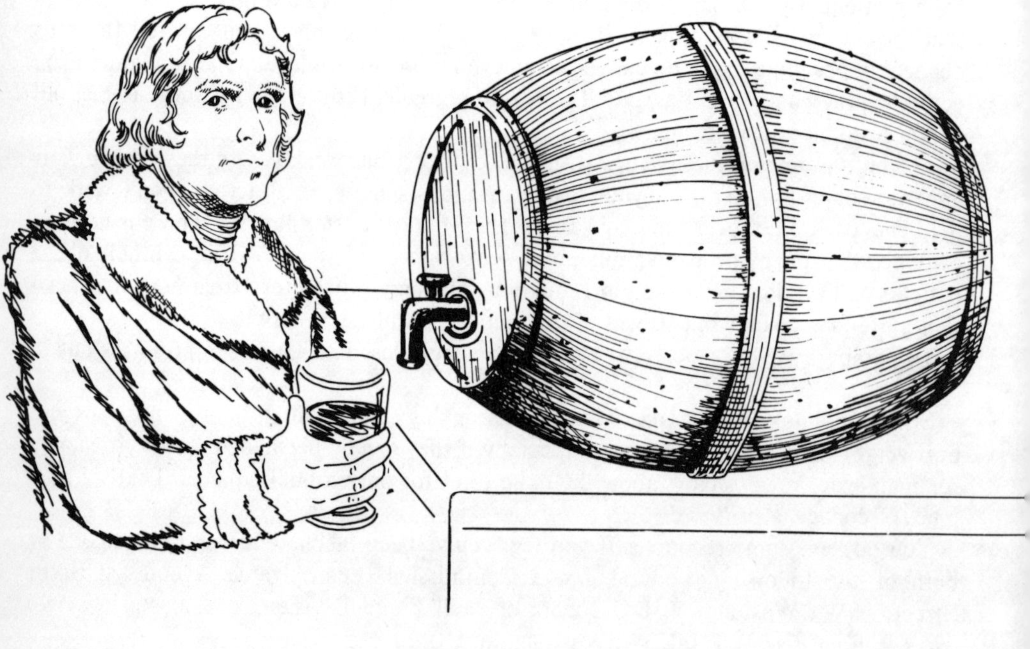

vidual they had ever met. He rode a horse from the time he could mount one until three days before he died. When he wasn't working in the government or striding through foreign courts, he was working in his garden, surveying, inventing, designing, or writing.

Jefferson arose at dawn, then wrote and read until breakfast. He had his major meal of the day at 3 P.M. after a hard ride. Then he worked until his light supper at 9 P.M. Usually he was in bed at 10 or 11 P.M.

He was almost a vegetarian. He wrote a friend: "I have lived temperately, eating little animal food and that not as an aliment so much as a condiment for the vegetables which constitute my principal diet." He believed one should always rise from the table a little bit hungry.

Jefferson was much more specific in 1819 when he prescribed the following diet for students at the University of Virginia.

Breakfast: No meat. Wheat or corn bread and butter. Milk or coffee au lait.

Dinner: "As great a variety of vegetables well cooked as you please." Soup. Meat (salt or fresh).

Supper: Corn or wheat bread. Milk or coffee au lait. No meat.

Such a diet yields 1,150 calories a day.

Jefferson also advised students to "drink at all times water, a young stomach needing no stimulating drinks, and the habit of using them being dangerous."

He drank water at least once a day. In addition, he wrote, "I double, however, the doctor's glass-and-a-half of wine, and even treble it with a friend, but half its effects by drinking weak wines only. The ardent wines I cannot drink, nor do I use ardent spirits in any form. Malt liquors and cider are my table drinks, and my breakfast . . . is of tea and coffee." Like George Washington, Jefferson was particularly fond of Madeira, and kept 12 gallons in his cellar at Monticello. He once called whisky "loathsome."

As for his meat eating, a friend wrote, "He never ate much hog-meat. He often told me, as I was giving out meat for the servants, that what I gave one of them for a week would be more than he would use in six months. He was especially fond of guinea fowls and for meat he preferred good beef, mutton, and lambs."

Alas, as Washington's Secretary of State, Jefferson contributed to his country's corpulence. He was the first to bring French cooks to the United States, and then first to use vanilla and macaroni in America. He brought from France recipes still used for nouilly a maccaroni, meringues, macaroons, ice cream, biscuit de Savoye, blanc mange, wine jellies, peches a l'eau, coffee, and for preserving green beans for winter. He also was the first President to serve dessert a la mode (with a ball of ice cream).

Because he was unhappy with the quality of Carolinian rice grown in America, he smuggled native rice out of the Piedmont district of Italy to grow at home—even though there was a death penalty attached to the exportation of rice from that area.

Jefferson was still lean and strong when he died in 1826 at the very decent age of 83. Unlike Washington, he had all his teeth; none was defective. His hazel-flecked gray eyes were still bright, although his sandy-red hair bore some gray. The illness characterized by an enlarged prostate took his life on the fiftieth anniversary of the signing of the Declaration of Independence he had authored.

Jefferson left a Canon for a Practical Life that every dieter should memorize: "We never repent of having eaten too little."

April — Week 3

This day shall be a memorial for you; so you must keep it as a feast to the Lord; through out your generations you must keep it as a perpetual ordinance. For seven days you must eat unleavened cakes; on the very first day you must clear your houses of leaven; for if anyone eats leavened bread from the first day to the seventh, that person shall be cut off from Israel.

EXODUS 12:15

You must observe this command; for it was on this very day that I brought you out of the land of Egypt.

EXODUS 12:17

Then the people bowed their heads in reverence. The Israelites went and did so; they did just as the Lord had commanded Moses and Aaron.

EXODUS 12:28

Now the first day of the feast of unleavened bread the disciples came to Jesus, saying unto Him, Where wilt thou that we prepare for thee to eat Passover?

MATTHEW 26:17

And the disciples did as Jesus had appointed them; and they made ready for the Passover.

MATTHEW 26:19

Now when the even was come, he sat down with the twelve.

MATTHEW 26:20

These quotes demonstrate the food connections of Passover and Easter, and how these feasts evoke your memories and emotions.

Anthropologically, these two holidays have agricultural roots. Early spring is the time when cows and ewes produce their new young. Ancient peoples offered their first fruit to higher powers they felt had favored them. Hence, the paschal sacrifice. It is also the first fruit offering of grain, hence the unleavened bread, or matzo. Easter is a word derived from the Anglo-Saxon word for spring, *Eostre*.

When Jesus sat down with his dozen followers to celebrate the Passover, he was obeying a commandment of God that Jews had observed since Moses proclaimed it back in the dark days of Egyptian slavery. Then, as now, the holiday was a celebration of redemption, of the rebirth of the Jewish people.

Since the Passover seder (ritual dinner) was the occasion of Christ's Last Supper, it also serves Christians, as the symbol of his sacrifice (the Lamb of God), and his resurrection, or passage through death to life.

Both Jews and Christians use food and wine to celebrate their spring holidays. For both religions, at this time, the egg is an important symbol of new life and resurrection. For both, too, the unleavened bread (matzos for Jews, wafers for Christians who take communion) is the symbol of reverence for him who provided.

Other foods at Passover and Easter have changed over the millennia. The main seder dish of lamb, served in the Land of Milk and Honey after the Exodus, was replaced by chicken in Europe and turkey in America. Among American Jews, the Passover dinner very much resembles the dinner served at the secular Thanksgiving holiday.

Among Christians, the most traditional main course for Easter is ham. While all manner of pork is specifically prohibited in the Old Testament chapter of Leviticus, interpretations of prohibitions change with the times.

This is all by way of pointing out how our spring religious celebrations have changed over the centuries. Despite the recitation of the events of the Exodus at seders and of the Resurrection at Easter Sunday services, most Jews and Christians use their respective April holidays as yet another excuse for dining and gorging.

Examining these modern celebrations can give a dieter some meaningful insights into the powerful cultural forces that drive eating urges. You need to look into your religious background (the same principle applies to Muslims, Hindus, Buddhists, etc.) to find the roots of your motivation to eat as a way of celebrating your faith.

At such celebrations as Passover and Easter, dieters are in trouble. Only the most militant can resist the call of the holiday banquet and hold back from the dishes of plenty served at the family table. Few dieters can resist this occasion as an important exception to their new eating plan and not leave the family table overstuffed.

Even if you are not at your parents' table, your deep-seated emotions impel you to dig in. Within you is the memory of yourself as a child at the family table, being urged to eat more. Inside you are the emotions, all mixed up, which make you feel, even today, that there is a direct proportion between how much you eat on this occasion and how much you show your mother, God, and Jesus that you love them.

Understanding these emotions is the first step toward untangling them. Once they are untangled—no small task—they can be dealt with, one by one. Then you can start dieting in earnest, secure in the knowledge that you can stay slim for the rest of your life. You will not permanently control your overeating until you take charge of the emotions behind that behavior.

As long as you use Passover, Easter, and every other celebration to gorge yourself, you will have a problem. As long as you use meals to express your love and assuage your feelings of guilt, you will have a problem. As long as you emotionally endow food, you will have a problem.

Still, you can observe religious holidays and every other celebration. Go back to the roots of the celebration. Revel in the reasons for its being. Consume the cultural and religious meanings. Express love for your mother, wife, or whoever prepared the meal by hugging, praising, and kissing, not by overeating.

Once you get a new perspective, you can observe holidays in every season. You can use traditional foods symbolically for religious purposes and not for emotional purposes that put and keep weight on.

Start now. Let Passover or Easter, whichever you observe, be a starting point, a rebirth, of a new you who will be slim and stay slim. Let this be the springtime of your new era of fitness.

April — Week 4

Now that spring is in full bloom, you should start planning for summer camp. There are diet camps for adults and for children, and now is the time to write away for details and applications.

While diet camps are not cheap, they offer some real advantages. You (or your child) live for a few weeks in an environment heavily devoted to physical fitness and weight loss. It can be a meaningful first step toward a lifetime of good eating and exercise habits. It provides a few weeks or months in the country to get your act together, counseled by people who can help you learn how to eat and exercise properly, and in the company of others who have a weight problem and want outdoor fun.

The fat-camp experience is a lot better than the diet-spa experience, in several ways. Spas are a few days or a week in a never-never land of sumptuous self-control. The feeling lingers only as long as the airplane flight home. Then you are back with the same old anxieties, same old nibbling, same old sloppy habits.

Summer camp is not exactly the real world either. But it is a lot closer, perhaps only a step or two away. The camper is better off. Lots more can be accomplished in terms of changing eating habits in the casual, informal, sweaty, down-to-earth atmosphere of camp than at a plush resort.

But before you shell out the significant fee, run down a simple checklist:

1. Is the camp's food plan well-rounded and calorie-controlled?

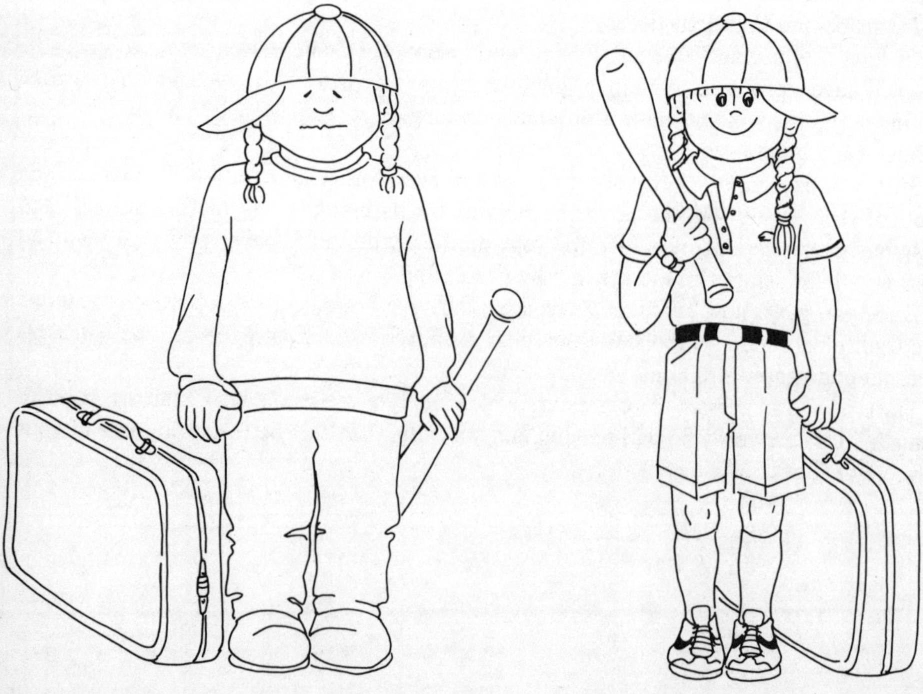

2. Is the camp supervised by a dietitian or nutritionist?
3. Does the camp have a medical director, either on site or close by?
4. Is the sports/exercise program integrated into every camper's daily activities?
5. Is the exercise program aerobic and strenuous enough to build up fitness?
6. Is it supervised by a qualified instructor with a degree in physical education or recreation?
7. Do campers learn good eating techniques that they can apply back home, in the real world?
8. Is there a regular program of behavior modification to help the camper convert bad eating habits into good ones?
9. Are there group sessions or counseling to help the camper take a look at himself or herself and better understand why he or she has been overeating?

The camp you seek should answer yes to all these questions.

You are probably aware that there are lots of sports and fitness camps vying for your dollars, from ultrafancy private camps to down-to-earth YMCA camps. While these camps will certainly increase your (or your child's) athletic skills and improve fitness, they will not necessarily reduce weight. Only a good diet program will do that.

Finally, there may be a tax write-off of the diet camp fee. Check with your accountant to see if you can deduct it under Ruling 55-261, as a medical expense for Health Institute Fees. You would need a prescription or statement from your own doctor saying the "treatments" at camp are necessary for the alleviation of a medical problem.

What follows is information on the best diet camps in the country.

Weight Watchers Camps
183 Madison Avenue
New York, NY 10016
Phone: (800) 223-5600 (in New York call collect 212-889-9500)

Like the food bearing the Weight Watchers imprimatur, these camps are licensed to other firms, in this case Campus Camping Corp. and Adult Camps Ltd.

There are seven WW camps for adults—defined as persons 19 years of age and older. They are located at Beloit College, Beloit, WI; Grand Lake Lodge, Lebanon, CT; East Stroudsburg, PA; Biscayne College, Miami, FL; University of Nevada, Las Vegas; University of Nevada, Reno; and Montreat-Anderson College, Montreat, NC. The camps in Connecticut, Florida, and Nevada are open year-round.

The minimum stay at these adult camps is one week. In addition, campers are allowed one free class per week in the fall at the WW group of their choice for every week spent at camp. There are no children at these camps.

The five kids' camps, for boys and girls 10-21 years, have four and seven-week sessions. The children's camps are at Carroll College, Waukesha, WI; Lakeland University, Sheboygan, WI; Lackawaxen in the Pocono Mountains of Pennsylvania; Appalachian State University, Asheville, NC; and Westmont College, Santa Barbara, CA. There is one girls-only camp located in Pennsburg, PA, near Valley Forge.

Camp Shane
Route 1, Box 48A
Ferndale, NY 12734
Phone: (914) 292-4644

Located 120 miles from Manhattan, Camp Shane follows the New York City Board of

Health Diet, one of the best ever constructed. Selma and Irving Ettenberg emphasize that "we own Camp Shane, we direct Camp Shane, and we live at camp all year." Theirs is unlike diet camps that rent facilities and hire different directors every year. Mrs. Ettenberg explained, "Our feelings are that children who have a weight problem generally go to food for their security. At camp, when that security is removed they need to have it replaced by tender loving care and attention that is readily available to them here."

Camp Shane is coed, for ages 7 to 17, and has three, six, and nine-week sessions. It also has special sessions for girls age 18 to 25.

Camp Del Mar
Suite D
8245 Ronson Road
San Diego, CA 92111
Phone collect: (714) 279-7800 (in California, 800-542-6005)

By the sea (what the camp name means in Spanish), overlooking the beaches of LaJolla, on the campus of the University of California at San Diego, this camp has unusually fine athletic facilities for boys, age 8 to 18.

"Many of our young men have a real interest in sports, but because of their weight, they have not been able to compete with others on the level they desire," explained camp director David Kempton. "The Del Mar boy finds that he can develop his sports interest and ability while losing weight."

Camp nutritionist Barbara Gunning (who is also a professor at California State University in San Diego) finds a 20- to 35-pound weight loss typical for a seven-week stay at Del Mar. She estimates that the average camper, fed a daily diet of 1,200 calories, works off 3,200 calories. The net loss of 2,000 calories a day results in a weight loss of about 4 pounds per week.

This camp is brother to Camp Murrietta for girls, both owned by Sportsworld.

Seascape
PO Box J
Brewster, MA 02631
Phone: (617) 389-2553 (business hours) or (617) 896-5479 (evenings, weekends)

Boasting a magnificent private facility on Cape Cod near the ocean, Seascape's objective is "permanent weight loss through nutrition education, physical activity, and development of new interests" for 100 girls 9 to 19 years old.

A quarter of a century old, it claims to be the original diet camp. Its owner, Dr. John A. Spargo, is a pediatrician and professor at Northeastern University. Camp nutritionist is Penelope S. Peckos, who was with Harvard and is now with Forsyth Dental Infirmary, Boston. The camp director is Patricia A. Goulding.

Seascape's diet is described as "high in protein, moderate in fat, and low in carbohydrates." Moreover, "each girl learns she can eat what everyone eats, but not as much and not as often."

Weight progress reports are sent to parents at midsummer and to parents and family physician at season's end.

Camp Murrieta
Suite D
8245 Ronson Road

San Diego, CA 92lll
Call collect: (714) 279-7800 (in California, 800-542-6005)

Actually, there are six Camp Murrietas for girls, located on college campuses in Wisconsin, Ohio, Virginia, Texas, California, and Washington state.

All campers get a 1,100-calorie daily diet, nutrition and cooking classes, and lots of aerobic exercise.

Young women 17 to 21 have a special program, with in-depth counseling and food preparation classes. A special four-week session is offered for 8 to 10 year olds.

Camelot
949 Northfield Road
Woodmere, NY 11598
Phone: (516) 374-0785

Camelot is actually eight different camps, five for girls, three for boys. Both boys and girls camp—separately, of course—at Southeastern Massachusetts University, near Cape Cod; at Susquehanna University, in Central Pennsylvania; and, at Whittier College in Southern California. Girls aged 10 to 17 and women aged 18 to 29 can also camp at the Camelots at the University of Wisconsin-LaCrosse and at Appalachian State University in the Blue Ridge Mountains of North Carolina.

Offered are full-summer sessions and 27-day sessions. The 1,200-calorie daily diet was designed by Morton B. Glenn, M.D., a noted New York physician-nutritionist who runs obesity clinics and was president of the American College of Nutrition. Darlyne Mostad, a registered dietitian, is the camp nutrition director. Dr. Glenn says, "Most of our campers have lost from 15 to 40 pounds in the camp season."

Camelot Camps are owned and run by the Hurwitz Family—mother Thelma, son Elliot, and daughter Michele and her husband Marc M. Friedman.

Kingsmont Camp
West Stockbridge, MA 01266
Phone: (413) 232-8518

Dr. Lloyd O. Appleton, the camp director, claims his campers lose 8,000 collective total pounds each summer. There are separate programs, staffs, and facilities for boys and girls age 7 to 18. There are four-week and eight-week sessions, which teach correct eating habits and offer lots of counseling with an emphasis on "developing self-confidence and a sense of belonging."

Camp Clover
Box 148
Mountaindale, NY 12763
Phone: (914) 434-2021

This camp for overweight girls admits campers as young as 6 years, according to the camp's director, Marcia J. Leff. There are four- and eight-week sessions.

Camp Mt. View
11-20 154 Street
Beechhurst, NY 11357
Phone: (212) 767-8998

This camp for girls, located in the Catskills, boasts individual losses of 5 to 40 pounds and 10 to 30 inches.

THE CAMELOT DIET
(10 DAY SAMPLE DAILY 1500 CALORIE MENUS)

SUNDAY

Strawberries
Cold Cereal or
 Poached Egg
Whole Wheat Toast
Skim Milk
Coffee/Sanka/Tea

Camelot Cheese
 Pizza
Salad Bar
Salad Dressing
Apple
Skim Milk
Iced Tea/Coffee

Snack:
Assorted Vegetables

Roast Beef au jus
Asparagus
Stewed Tomatoes
Salad Bar
Salad Dressing
Orange Frappe
Iced Tea/Coffee

Evening Snack:
Fruit

MONDAY

Orange Juice
Cold Cereal or
French Toast
Skim Milk
Coffee/Sanka/Tea

Tuna Salad in Lettuce,
 Sliced Tomato
Assorted Relish

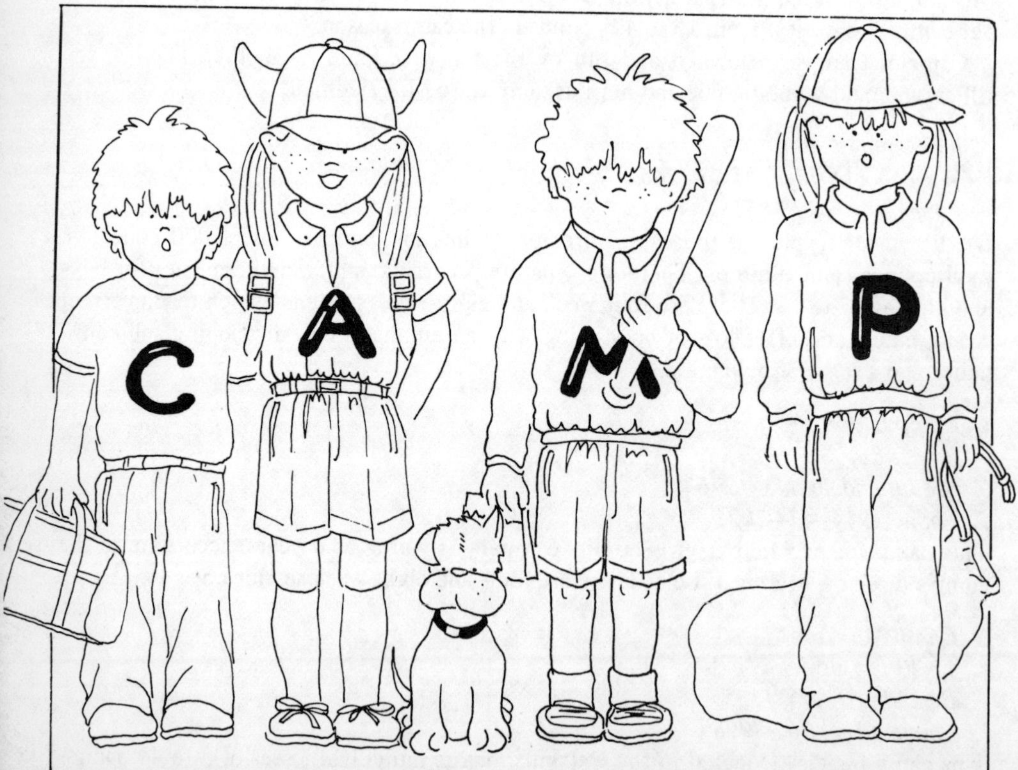

Rye Krisp
Nectarine
Skim Milk
Iced Tea/Coffee

Snack:
Assorted Vegetables

Low Calorie Cranberry Juice
Polynesian Chicken
Spring Garden Peas
Celery with Caraway Seed
Chilled Melon
Iced Tea/Coffee

Evening Snack:
Popcorn

TUESDAY

½ Banana
Cold Cereal or
  Oatmeal/Cinnamon
Skim Milk
Coffee/Sanka/Tea

Sloppy Joe on Bun
Salad Bar
Salad Dressing
Fresh Peach
Skim Milk
Iced Tea/Coffee

Snack:
Assorted Vegetables

Baked Halibut,
  Italian Style
Green Beans
Cole Slaw
Ice Cream
Iced Tea/Lemonade/
  Coffee

Evening Snack:
Cinnamon Tea
2 Graham Crackers

WEDNESDAY

Grapefruit Sections
Cold Cereal or
  Melted Cheddar
  Cheese on Raisin Toast
Skim Milk
Coffee/Sanka/Tea

Tomato Juice
Chicken Salad
Carrot/Celery Sticks
Seasoned Rye Krisp
Fresh Plums
Skim Milk
Iced Tea/Coffee

Snack:
Assorted Vegetables

Veal Scallopine with garlic,
  mushrooms, oregano, tomato sauce,
Baked Squash, Lettuce Wedge
Camelot 1000 Is. Dressing
Lemon Snow
Iced Tea/Coffee

Evening Snack:
Fruit

THURSDAY

Quartered Orange
Cold Cereal or
  Soft or hard cooked Egg
Whole Wheat Toast
Skim Milk
Coffee/Sanka/Tea

Chef Salad:
  Swiss Cheese
  Turkey
  Beef
  Vegetable Garnish
  Sl. Tomato
  Radishes
  Asparagus, Greens,
Seasoned Rye Krisp
Ice Cream
Iced Tea/Coffee

Snack:
Assorted Vegetables

Broiled Steak
Broccoli
Broiled Tomatoes
Salad Bar
Salad Dressing
Baked Apple
Iced Tea/coffee

Evening Snack:
Fresh Fruit

FRIDAY

Applesauce
Cold Cereal or
Toasted English Muffin
Poached Egg and
Cheese Sauce
Skim Milk
Coffee/Sanka/Tea

California Fruit Plate
Cottage Cheese
Waverly Wafers
Skim Milk
Strawberries
Iced Tea/Coffee

Snack:
Assorted Vegetables

Cook-Out:
B-B-Q Chicken
½ Corn on the Cob
Assorted Vegetables (raw)
Chilled Watermelon
Cold Drinks

Evening Snack:
Cinnamon Tea

SATURDAY

Orange Juice
Cold Cereal or
Cream of Wheat
Skim Milk
Coffee/Sanka/Tea

Zesty Taco
Salad Bar
Salad Dressing
Apple
Skim Milk
Iced Tea/Coffee

Snack:
Assorted Vegetables

Hawaiian Fish
Kabobs Teriyaki
Lemon Mint Beans
Chopped Spinach
Salad Bar
Salad Dressing
Ice Cream
Iced Tea/Coffee

Evening Snack:
Fresh Fruit

SUNDAY

Blueberries
Cold Cereal or
Cottage Cheese
Cinnamon Toast
Skim Milk
Coffee/Sanka/Tea

Reuben Sandwich (Turkey/Cheese
Sauerkraut on Rye)
Marinated Bean Salad
Orange
Skim Milk
Iced Tea/Coffee

Snack:
Assorted Vegetables

Pineapple Frappe
Beef Stroganoff
Rice
Pickled Beets
Salad Bar
Salad Dressing
Pear
Iced Tea/Coffee

Evening Snack:
Popcorn

MONDAY

½ Grapefruit
Cold Cereal or
Baked Egg au Gratin
Wheat Toast
Skim Milk
Coffee/Sanka/Tea

Cheeseburger
½ Hamburger Roll
Sliced Onion
Sliced Tomatoes
Lettuce
Mustard
Apple
Skim Milk
Iced Tea/Coffee

Snack:
Assorted Vegetables

Roast Turkey
Baked Squash
Parsley Carrots
Salad Bar
Salad Dressing
Pineapple Chunks
Iced Tea/Coffee

Evening Snack:
Fresh Fruit

TUESDAY

½ Banana
Cold Cereal or Toasted Bagel
Whipped Neufchatel
Hard Cooked Egg
Skim Milk
Coffee/Sanka/Tea

Trip Day:

Chicken Sandwich
Whole Wheat Bread
Mustard
Lettuce
Dill Pickle
Carrot/Celery Sticks
Fresh Peach
Cold Drinks

Snack:
Ice Cream on Trip

Cheesey Fish Fillets
Broccoli/Lemon Wedge
Zucchini-Italian style
Salad Bar
Salad Dressing
Chilled Melon
Iced Tea/Coffee

Evening Snack:
Hot Tea or Coffee

CAMELOT for Boys
949 Northfield Rd.,
Woodmere, New York 11598
Phone: (516) 374-0785

May — Week 1

Hurray, hurray, it's the first of May!

Earnest dieting starts today.

It's a fact that more people begin diets in May than in any other month. Yes, many resolve to lose weight on New Year's Day, but May is more urgent, with its longer days of warm sunshine reminding us that we will soon be on the beach, at the pool, or on the cycle or jogging path in scant, revealing clothes.

This time you should start at "Go" and all fresh. Now that you are "psyched up," you need to start the right eating habits, start exercising, and start on an effective and safe diet.

The right diet is one you lose weight on. At the same time it is safe enough to serve you for the rest of your life. That rules out fad diets.

Here are ten questions that will help you evaluate any diet regimen you plan to follow:

1. *Does the diet provide adequate protein—at least 44 grams a day if you are female, 56 grams if you are male?*

It should. Protein gets its name from the Greek word for "first" because it is the number-one nutrient. Watch out for faddish vegetarian and near-vegetarian diets that exclude animal and fish products or allow only minuscule amounts. The same caution applies to high-carbohydrate diets (such as the rice diet), fruit diets, and high-fat diets (such as the whipped cream diet). Your body requires protein for body maintenance and repair, for the production of most hormones, and for its fight against germs.

2. *Does the diet provide adequate carbohydrates—at least 60 grams a day?*

If you have cut back on daily calories and are starting to "burn" body fat, you'll need a minimum of carbohydrates in food to prevent a condition known as *ketosis.* Besides causing bad breath, ketosis can cause complications in some people, especially pregnant women and those with diabetes and gout. It is called ketosis because in breaking down fats for energy, the body makes by-products known as ketones. You can tell if you are in ketosis with a simple urine test or a *Ketostix* that you can purchase in the drugstore.

3. *Does the diet provide no more than a third of the calories as fat, with at least half as polyunsaturated fats?*

About 30 percent of your daily calories from fats and oils is the limit, because a high-fat diet is generally unhealthy. Also, polyunsaturated fats are better for your heart and arteries than saturated fats. Here's how to tell the difference. "Bad" saturated fats are solid at room temperature (coconut oil, butter, lard, hydrogenated oil), and "good" polyunsaturated fats are liquid at room temperature (soy oil, safflower oil, corn oil).

4. *Does the diet emphasize one kind of food to the exclusion of most, or all others?*

If so, watch out. Human beings are omnivores, which means we are neither exclusively meat eaters (carnivores) nor plant eaters (herbivores). Nor can we exist on fruit alone, which some diets specify. Every day you need to eat foods from the four food groups: protein (meat, eggs, nuts, legumes); dairy (milk, yogurt, cheeses); vegetables and fruits; breads and grains. Well-rounded diets are not only healthier, but they are more durable. This applies to vegetarian diets as well.

5. *Is the diet less than 1,000 calories a day?*

If so, make sure you are under a doctor's care and are taking vitamin-mineral supplements because you won't get enough of these micronutrients in so little food. Be wary of hucksters who want to sell you powders to mix with milk or water that supply "all" the nutrition you need.

6. *Is the diet based on a secret no one has discovered before?*
There are no secrets in dieting. Don't trust anyone who tells you he or she has one. Here's the only secret: You can lose weight on *any* diet. The questions are these: For how long? How safely?

7. *Has the diet been scientifically evaluated by reputable nutritionists, physicians, or both?*
Be wary of new diets unless they have been tried on hundreds or thousands of overweight people and by researchers other than the "discoverer." The results should have been objectively compared to the results of a similar number of persons on other diets or on no diets. All data should have been published in reputable scientific journals. If none of these apply to your diet, you're being fed hogwash.

8. *What kind of scientific reputation has the originator or author of the diet?*
You're looking for an excellent scientific reputation in medical and nutritional circles. Simply being a physician or other kind of doctor doesn't qualify. The author of the diet should have a deep knowledge of nutrition and some experimental and clinical experience, and should have published many reports of his or her work in scientific and medical journals. Unfortunately, lots of fast-buck artists with advanced degrees fabricate diets based on outrageous pet theories of no substance and no validity.

9. *Is someone making lots of money with this diet—either the author of a book or the supplier of some drug or nutrient?*
Everyone in the publishing business is looking for a doctor-writer twosome to make a fortune by writing a fad-diet book. The crazier the gimmick, the better. Alas, there are no new truths in dieting. The durable truths are free and waiting to be used. Fad-diet book authors work hard to persuade you otherwise. Ditto the makers of vitamins, supplements, and other "magic" pills to "melt" the fat off.

10. *Is the diet recommended by a weight-reducing group?*

Your best bet is to join a good group like Weight Watchers, Diet Workshop, TOPS, or Overeaters Anonymous. You probably need both the discipline of attending meetings and the support of others like you. Millions of dieters belong to groups. They find solace there, as well as support, good advice, and a program that works.

May — Week 2

D is for daily diet.

But before you take up any scheme to lose weight, know what basic nutrients you need in your daily diet.

Protein is first because that's what the name means, but the protein you eat every day has to be of the right quality and the right quantity.

Protein varies in quality. The highest-quality protein you can eat comes from animals and their products. Egg white, or albumin, is the best and considered the reference protein by nutritionists. Caseine, the protein of milk and milk products, is nearly as high in quality. Protein in meat, that is, the muscles of animals (including fish), is also of very high quality. However, the protein of gelatin is low quality. Lowest of all is protein from most plants.

The quality of a protein is based on its content of amino acids. Every bit of protein you eat is broken down by your body to these chemical components. Then the body reassembles the amino acids to make the proteins it needs for new cells, hormones, and other uses.

Your body makes many of the amino acids it requires, but eight important ones cannot be made and so must be obtained from food. A further problem is that your body cannot store amino acids. All the amino acids obtained in food are used immediately, in the proportions the body needs. Amino acids that don't fulfill these proportions are stripped down still further and transformed into sugar.

If you are going on a vegetarian diet, you have to mix your nuts, cereals, and grains so that you get these amino acids in the proper balance. It can be done, but you have to know what you are doing.

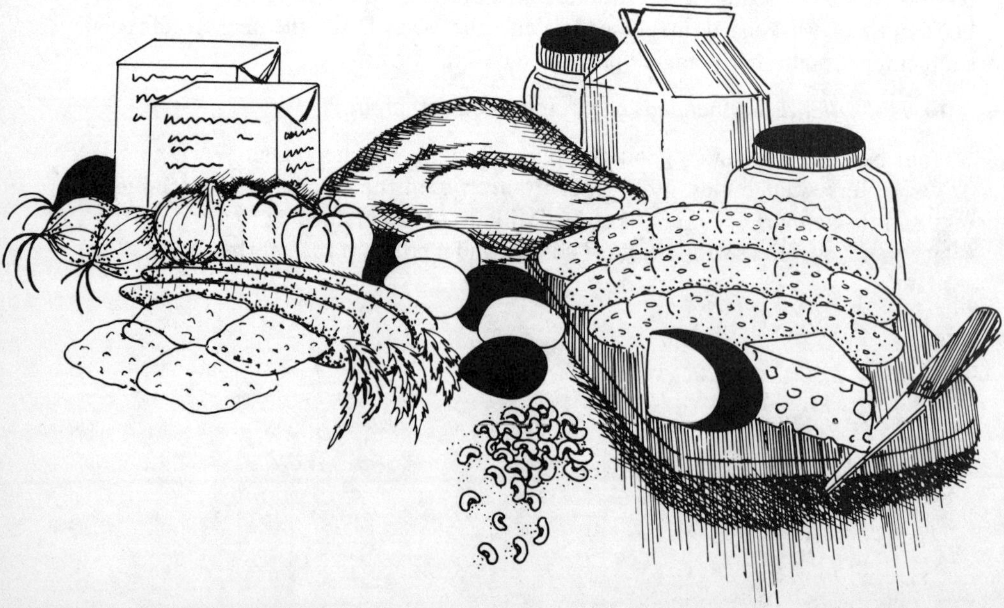

Here are the daily amino acid needs of a 154-pound person: isoleucine, 0.84 grams; leucine, 1.12 g; lysine, 0.84 g; methionine, 0.7 g; phenylalanine, 0.98 g; threonine, 0.56 g; tryptophan, 0.21 g; and valine, 1.12 g.

Peanuts are deficient in methionine, but wheat has an excess—that's how a peanut butter sandwich gives you complete protein. Incidentally, gelatin is also deficient in this amino acid, which is why so many dieters who tried to live on "liquid protein" made from gelatin got into nutritional difficulties.

If you want to diet the vegetarian way, follow Frances Moore Lappe's safe way in *Diet for a Small Planet* (Ballantine, 1982), or contact the Seventh Day Adventists at Box 75, Loma Linda, CA 92354. Beware of diets that tell you to eat only leafy vegetables and fresh fruits, or only grapefruit, or only rice, or any one food that is low in protein.

According to the National Academy of Sciences, if you eat a very high quality protein such as egg white, you need only about 33 grams a day (for a 154-pound person). But since most people get their protein from a variety of sources, the NAS recommends about 44 grams for women, 56 grams a day for men.

All the protein you eat in excess of your body's needs is converted to glucose, the main source of energy in the body. This same fate is met by all the starches and other carbohydrates you eat. (So much for the value of high-protein diets.)

The problem with eating sugar is that it enters the blood stream within minutes. This gives you a "high." Coffee causes this same high by provoking the liver to release glucose, the main sugar of the body. The body copes with this by issuing the hormone insulin to bring the sugar level down to normal. This quick rise and fall of blood sugar, or "spiking," causes hunger pangs in the morning after a sweet roll or glazed doughnut. The body takes longer to digest starches and other complex carbohydrates and convert them to sugar. That's why a bowl of breakfast cereal holds off hunger better than a danish for breakfast.

Whatever sugar the body doesn't burn gets stored, either as the body starch known as glycogen, in liver and muscles, or as fat under the belly and under the skin—especially on breasts, buttocks, and thighs. Much of the fat in food also gets stored. In a pinch, some of it can be burned as a secondary source of energy.

Protein, carbohydrate, and fat are the three major nutrients you need every day. You also need vitamins A, B-complex, C, D, E, and tiny amounts of such minerals as calcium, phosphorus, and zinc. Altogether you need about 50 dietary chemicals to stay healthy and function well. (See the guide to vitamins and minerals at the back of this book for more information.)

Of course, you can get many vitamins and minerals (often called micronutrients) in pill form. But an even better way is to follow a rounded diet. That means eating a variety of foods in the five major groups. It takes at least 1,200 calories a day to get all these.

Any diet that does not include foods from the protein group (eggs, meat, nuts, legumes, cereals); dairy group (milk, cheeses, yogurt); vegetable group; fruit group; and grains and breads is shortchanging you.

Sure, you'll lose weight on a one-food diet. But you may lose your health as well.

The best way, the only way, to lose weight is to go on a diet that will take off pounds safely and keep them off. This is a diet you can live on for life. Crash diets are worse than temporary; they are dangerous.

May — Week 3

I is for Integrity.

If you are going to lose weight, you need to go on—and stay on—a diet that has integrity.

That precludes fad diets, like the best-selling diet books of the past and present. It means a diet that you can marry—one that you will live with and be faithful to for the rest of your life. Any diet short of these goals will sooner or later fail.

The most effective and safest diets offer meal plans for you to follow. They allow options and substitutes which you select from lists. Because these diets allow you to exchange one food on a list for another, they are called "exchange diets."

The grandaddy of exchange diets is that developed for diabetics by the American Diabetic Association and the American Dietetic Association. The late Dr. Norman Jolliffe of the New York City Health Department adapted and refined this diet to come up with his Prudent Diet. This, in turn, was adapted by Weight Watchers, Diet Workshop, and other dieting organizations.

A diet with integrity gives you:

- Enough calories to live on, but few enough calories to lose weight with. For most people, that's about 1,200 calories a day.
- A minimum of 60 grams of protein; a maximum 30 percent of calories in fat, half of those as polyunsaturated fat; and the rest of the calories from carbohydrates, particularly the complex carbohydrates in breads and cereals, vegetables, and fruit.
- No more than 300 milligrams a day of cholesterol and 5 grams a day of salt.
- An adequate amount of roughage, or fiber.
- Proper portions of food from all five food groups: protein, dairy, grains and cereals, vegetables, and fruits.

What follows is a diet that has Integrity with a capital *I*. It is the original 1,200-calorie New York City diet—durable, safe, effective, and simple enough to master and memorize. (Do not confuse this diet with the inferior *I Love New York Diet*).

Breakfast

For fruit that's high in vitamin C, choose one: ½ medium grapefruit, ½ medium mango, ½ medium cantaloupe, 1 medium orange, 1 cup strawberries, 1 large tangerine, 8 ounces tomato juice or 4 ounces orange or grapefruit juice.

For protein food, choose one: 2 ounces cottage or pot cheese, 1 ounce hard cheese, 2 ounces cooked or canned fish, or 1 egg.

For bread or cereal, whole grain or enriched, choose one: 1 slice bread, ¾ cups ready-to-eat cereal, or ½ cup cooked cereal.

8 ounces skim milk.

Coffee or tea.

Lunch

For protein food, choose one: 2 ounces fish, poultry or lean meat, 4 ounces cottage cheese, 2 ounces hard cheese, 1 egg, or 2 level tablespoons peanut butter.

For bread, 2 slices of whole grain or enriched bread.

Raw or cooked vegetables, except potatoes, peas, corn, beans, rice, and grits.

For fruit, single serving, choose one: 1 medium apple or peach; 2 to 3 apricots, prunes or plums; 1 small banana or pear; ½ cup berries; 4 ounces grapes or cherries; ½ small honeydew; ½ cup pineapple; 2 tablespoons raisins; or ½ round slice watermelon.

Coffee or tea.

Dinner

For protein food, choose one: 4 ounces cooked fish, poultry, or lean meat.

A high-in-vitamin-A vegetable such as broccoli, carrots, chicory, escarole, mustard greens, collard, pumpkin, winter squash, spinach, or watercress.

A potato or ½ cup peas or corn, 1 small ear fresh corn, ½ cup beans, ½ cup cooked rice, ½ cup cooked spaghetti, ½ cup cooked macaroni, ½ cup sweet potato or yams, ½ cup cooked grits, or ½ cup green lima beans.

Other vegetables you may eat freely include asparagus, broccoli, Brussels sprouts, carrots, cauliflower, celery, cucumber, dandelion greens, escarole, kale, green beans, lettuce, mushrooms, mustard greens, parsley, romaine lettuce, spinach, summer squash, tomatoes, and turnip greens.

For fruit, single serving, choose one: 1 medium apple or peach; 2 to 3 apricots, prunes, or plums; 1 small banana or pear; ½ cup berries; 4 ounces grapes or cherries; ½ small honeydew; ½ cup pineapple; 2 tablespoons raisins; or ½ round slice watermelon.

Coffee or tea.

Other Daily Foods

Fats (three servings daily from following): 2 teaspoons french dressing, 1 teaspoon vegetable oil margarine, 1 teaspoon mayonnaise, or 1 teaspoon vegetable oil.

Milk: 2 cups skim or buttermilk or 1 cup evaporated milk or ⅔ cup nonfat dry milk solids.

Foods to Avoid

Bacon, fatty meats, sausage, beer, liquor, wines, butter, margarine (other than what's allowed above), cakes, candies, crackers, doughnuts, pastries, pies, cookies, chocolates, nuts, whipping cream, sour cream, cream cheese, nondairy cream substitutes, french fries, potato chips, pizza, popcorn, pretzels and similar snack foods, gelatin desserts, puddings (sugar-sweetened), gravies and sauces, honey, jams, jellies, sugar and syrup, ice cream, ices, ice milk, sherbets, whole milk, muffins, pancakes, waffles, olives, sugar-sweetened soda, fruit-flavored yogurt.

May — Week 4

E is for exercise.

It can help you lose fat, firm up the sagging flesh left behind, and put you in a slimming frame of mind.

To lose a pound, you have to expend an *extra* 3,500 calories beyond what you expend now, and eat no more calories. That's jogging 4 hours and 15 minutes on level ground at 5 mph, or swimming the crawl at 2 mph for 2 hours and 11 minutes, or climbing stairs for 6 hours and 56 minutes.

Now, your body doesn't care over what period of time this occurs. So, if over five days you jogged 51 minutes a day, or swam 26 minutes a day, or climbed stairs for 1 hour and 23 minutes a day, you would still lose a pound. If you cut back on the calories you eat, as you increase the calories you expend through physical activities, you can lose weight even more rapidly.

Dr. Frank Konishi of Southern Illinois University, Carbondale, has compiled charts that show how you can do this. They are in his book, *Exercise Equivalent of Food*, published by his university's press. He shows how you can lose 15 pounds a month by walking, cycling, swimming, or jogging an hour a day—*if* you also cut back your diet by 1,000 calories a day. Or, you can lose that 15 pounds in two months by exercising only half an hour a day and cutting back by 600 calories.

Because diet and exercise work hand-in-glove to accomplish a trim, firm figure, Weight Watchers added Pepstep to its program. Diet Workshop has had an exercise program for years, and aerobic dancing and Jazzercise have captured many thousands of female followers.

Because it helps your body increase its expenditure of calories, exercise helps reduce fat all over your body. The problem is that the fat on your body is not equally distributed. There is more fat on your rump than on your ribs. And there are individual variations. That's what makes one woman more bosomy than another. Breasts are mostly fat. Except during times of breast feeding, the milk glands are very small.

Many men have a tendency to accumulate fat in their lower abdomen and develop "pot bellies," especially in middle age. The tendency is inherited, but the fat accumulation is strictly from overeating.

Gyms and health clubs make many claims about altering fat accumulation by spot reducing, but the truth is that exercise can selectively reduce the fat on only two areas of the body: the tummy and the back, where relatively broad layers of fat overlay large flat muscles.

Also, some kinds of exercises actually serve to increase the girth of limbs and waist. After all, weight lifters build up muscles with exercise.

So be sure you exercise properly, or you won't slim down.

The best slimming exercises are repetitive rather than resistant. That means doing lots of the same exercise every day. Of course, it's boring—but it works.

(This is all explained in detail in the *Dieter's Almanac* Exercise Plan in the beginning of this book. If you get started on the three-month plan now, you'll be a lot firmer and stronger by the first of August. And your physical endurance will be greater, too.)

Here are specifics about the number of calories your favorite sport burns up per minute. They are taken from from *The Fitness Fact Book* by Theodore Berland (Newspaper Enterprise Association, 1980).

CALORIE USE TABLE

Activity	Calories per minute
Jogging-running (16 mph on level ground)	65.2
Swimming (sidestroke at 2 mph)	50.0
Jogging-running (15 mph on level ground)	48.0
Swimming (backstroke at 2 mph)	33.3
Swimming (breast stroke at 2 mph)	30.8
Swimming (crawl at 2 mph)	26.7
Rowing (12 mph)	25.0
Snowshoeing (on level snow with 44-lb. load)	20.2
Football-soccer	16.1
Skiing (cross-country at 7.5 mph on level snow)	15.8
Jogging-running (7 mph up 8.6% grade)	15.8
Skiing (cross-country uphill)	15.6
Jogging-running (10 mph on level ground)	15.0
Jogging-running (5 mph on level ground)	13.7
Wrestling	13.2
Skating (roller at 13 mph)	13.0
Walking (in 12-15 in. of level snow)	12.7
Walking (3.5 mph up 14.4% grade)	12.3
Handball-squash-racketball (competitive)	12.0
Rope skipping (120-170 turns per minute)	12.0
Skiing (cross-country at 5 mph on level snow)	12.0
Calisthenics (parallel-bar gymnastics)	11.8
Sculling (3.5 mph)	11.2
Basketball (competitive)	11.0
Cycling (13 mph on level ground)	11.0
Rowing (3.5 mph)	11.0
Walking (in 2.5 in. of level snow)	10.7
Snowshoeing (2.5 mph on level snow with no load)	10.3
Handball-squash-racquetball (social)	10.5
Climbing (mountain)	10.0
Skiing (downhill at 10 mph)	10.0
Stair climbing (165-lb. person)	9.8
Horseback riding (gallop, posting)	9.5
Walking (3.5 mph up 8.6% grade)	9.3
Swimming (sidestroke at 1 mph)	9.2
Basketball (social)	9.0
Calisthenics (deep knee bends)	9.0
Calisthenics (push-ups)	9.0
Canoeing (5 mph)	9.0
Paddleball	9.0
Skiing (cross-country at 3 mph on level snow)	9.0
Stair climbing (152-lb. person)	8.4
Swimming (backstroke at 1 mph)	8.3
Climbing (hill)	8.2
Skiing (water)	8.0
Skating (roller at 9 mph)	7.8
Walking (4.6 mph on level ground)	7.8
Tennis (singles)	7.5
Badminton (competitive)	7.5
Walking (3.5 mph up 5.5% grade)	7.5
Walking (2.4 mph up 8.6% grade)	7.2
Dancing (rhumba, disco or square dance)	7.0
Golf (pulling cart or carrying bag)	7.0
Sculling (3 mph)	7.0
Swimming (crawl at 1 mph)	7.0
Swimming (breast stroke at 1 mph)	6.8
Skating (hockey or ice skating at 10 mph)	6.6
Baseball-softball (pitching)	6.5
Calisthenics (side straddle hop)	6.5
Canoeing (4 mph)	6.5
Horseback riding (trot, posting)	6.5
Sculling (2.5 mph)	6.4
Golf (walking with caddie)	6.2
Tennis (doubles)	6.0
Stair climbing (130-lb. person)	6.0
Walking (2.3 mph up 5.5% grade)	5.8
Volleyball (competitive)	5.8
Dancing (waltz)	5.7
Dancing (fox trot)	5.5
Badminton (social)	5.5
Cycling (10 mph on level ground)	5.3
Fencing	5.0
Golf (using wood)	5.0
Table tennis	5.0
Rowing (2.5 mph)	5.0
Walking (3.5 mph on level ground)	4.8
Walking (2.5 mph up 5% grade)	4.8
Calisthenics (leg raises)	4.8
Dancing (Petronella)	4.7
Baseball-softball (fielding)	4.7
Horseback riding (trot, sitting)	4.5
Walking (2 mph up 5% grade)	4.2
Billiards	3.9
Canoeing (2.5 mph)	3.8
Golf (using iron)	3.7
Calisthenics (trunk exercises)	3.5
Walking (2.3 mph on level ground)	3.5
Volleyball (social)	3.5
Cycling (5.5 mph on level ground)	3.2
Calisthenics (abdominal exercises)	3.0
Golf (using power cart or putting)	3.0
Horseback riding (walk, sitting)	3.0
Bowling	2.5
Calisthenics (balancing exercises)	2.5
Driving	2.0
Standing	1.5
Lying down	1.5
Sleeping	1.1

May — Week 5

T is for training.

Diet and exercise are not enough. To lose weight and keep it off—the primary goal of the slimming job you're undertaking—you also have to train yourself in new, slimming ways. This means developing new habits—regular practices of proper eating and exercising. In other words, you have to modify your behavior.

Of course, there are emotional reasons for such fattening behavior as nibbling in the kitchen or cramming sweets into your mouth. Psychotherapy can find out these reasons. But you don't have to know the reasons underlying your behavior to change it. Instead, you can apply the techniques of behavior modification. These techniques are so successful that the big diet clubs—Weight Watchers, Diet Workshop, TOPS, and Overeaters Anonymous—teach them to their members.

Dr. Albert J. Stunkard of the University of Pennsylvania found in a study of TOPS dieters that those who followed their club's rules *and* modified their behavior were much more successful at losing weight than were members who merely followed the rules.

You are better off learning to modify your behavior in one of these groups. But you can teach yourself to develop good new habits to replace the bad old ones. There are good instructions in two books: *Act Thin, Stay Thin* by Dr. Richard Stuart (Norton, 1978) and *Eating Is Okay* by Drs. Henry A. Jordan, Leonard S. Levitz, and Gordon Kimbrell (New American Library, 1977).

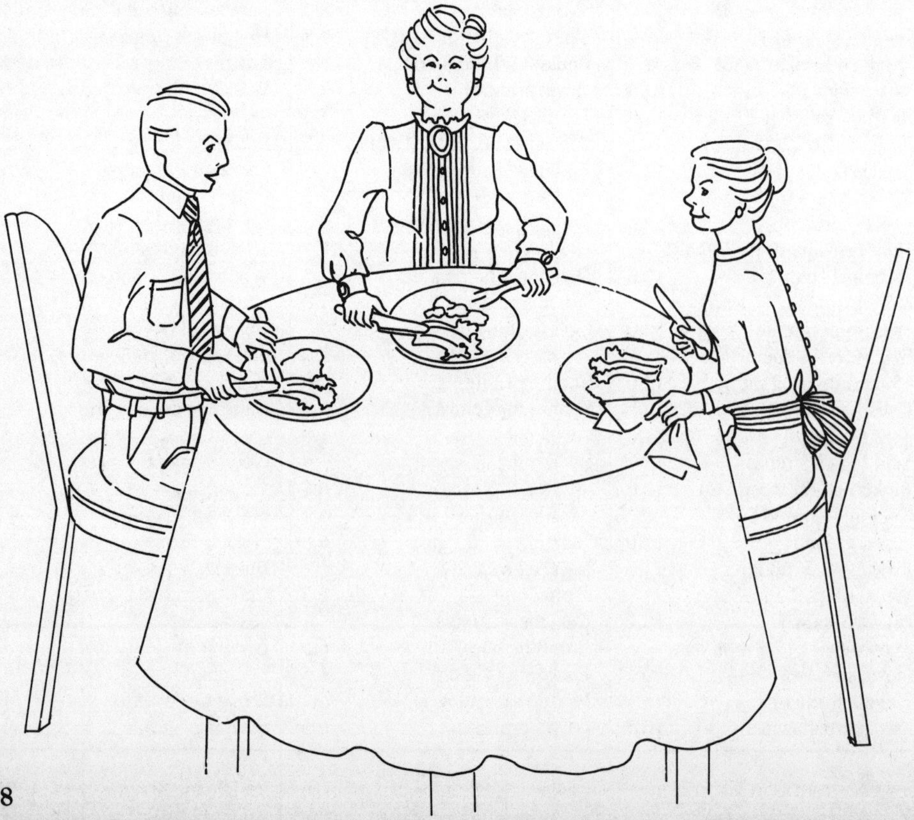

Dr. Stuart, of the University of Utah and psychology director of Weight Watchers International, points out that overweight people eat too fast; they have to learn to slow down. He quotes studies showing that people who eat slowly are less hungry than those who eat quickly, even though both kinds of eaters eat exactly the same amounts of food.

He advises you to eat slowly enough to appreciate the taste and smell and texture of food. You should be able to feel the tomato seeds on your tongue, smell the distinct aroma of cooked eggs, taste the saltiness of rare steak. He suggests you follow this regimen at your main meal of the day:

1. When you sit down at the table with others, leave the utensils on the table for the first two minutes of the meal, as you think quietly to yourself about how you will work on slowing down the rate of your eating.

2. Before you start to eat, cut the food on your plate into small bite-sized portions.

3. Pick up your fork and put one portion in your mouth, putting the fork back down on the plate as soon as it is empty.

4. Chew the food carefully, even thoughtfully. Feel the texture of the food with your tongue as it is ground into smaller morsels by your teeth. Try to sense its saltiness or sweetness, its bitterness or sourness. Concentrate on smelling its aroma. Focus your attention on the experience of eating so that you can capture its full enjoyment.

5. When the food has been swallowed, join in the conversation. Say something before picking up your fork for another bite. This next forkful will again become the focus of your attention.

6. Make certain that you are the *last* person to start eating each new course as it is served. Do this in order to extend to its maximum the length of time you spend eating your meal.

Jordan, Levitz, and Kimbrell of the University of Pennsylvania suggest that you carefully plan your day's eating activities as a way of curbing your impulsive eating. They suggest the following:

- Plan a short delay before starting to eat.
- Swallow the food in your mouth before picking up more with your utensils.
- Plan a series of brief delays during meals and snacks by:
  (1) putting down utensils,
  (2) sipping a beverage,
  (3) using a napkin more frequently,
  (4) engaging in a conversation.
- Keep extra food away from the table. This means keeping platters in the kitchen.
- When food platters are on the table, pass them away from you.
- Use measuring spoons and cups to serve the food in controlled portions.
- Eat preferred food first, not "best for last."
- Always leave a small amount of food on your plate.
- Clear the table immediately after each course. If this is not possible, remove or move your own plate from your place.
- Cover your plate with your napkin as a signal to yourself that the meal has ended.
- Have someone else remove, store, or throw away leftovers if these are a problem for you.

Losing weight is not easy, but it can be done.

You *can* do it. You can also keep the weight off with new eating habits. Now is the time to start to develop these habits.

June — Week 1

Don't be too surprised if your priest, minister, or rabbi starts pushing exercise. After all, the body is the temple of the soul. There are Jog for Jesus classes, and Passover Push-Ups groups. And that's just the beginning. There are also the Damascus Walk and the Bar Mitzvah Bounce. Exercise programs work in congregant groups, according to a participant, "because I could cheat on a diet but I couldn't cheat on Jesus."

Whether your motivation is religious or not, the beginning of June, with its lengthening glorious days, is the time to get started on your outdoor exercise program. (If you have completed the *Dieter's Almanac* Exercise Plan, you should be in shape to start now. If not, get started on this three-month program as soon as you can. If you begin now, you'll be in top shape for Labor Day, when the days are still long and warm.)

You may feel that because you are on the go all day, you don't need to exercise. But being on your feet all day in a store, office, or factory is not the same as jogging or fast walking. Sure, your feet may hurt, but working on your feet doesn't get up your heart and breathing rates to the point where you sweat. That's the point you want to reach and want to maintain. The American College of Sports Medicine suggests that if you are on a diet, you should expend at least 300 calories for 20 minutes, three times a week, in some form of exercise (900 total calories a week). Or you can work out four times a week for 20 minutes, expending only 200 calories per session (800 total calories).

Any exercise program below this level of activity will take no fat from your body. Even a 1,000-calorie-a-week exercise program, which is slightly above the recommended basement level, will take off but a quarter of a pound of fat a week.

Exercise expert Reed Humphrey of the Human Energy Research Laboratory at the University of Pittsburgh recommends that you start out by keeping an exercise diary. This is essentially a daily calendar on which you record the type of exercise and the time spent doing it. If you didn't exercise that day, you should note the reason for the abstinence.

In general, Humphrey notes in an article in *Obesity-Bariatric Medicine*, "group exercise is preferred over individual home-based exercise. Attrition rates are much lower in group programs. This may be related to the camaraderie that develops among patients which acts as a reinforcement for personal commitment."

Dr. Robert E. Leach, chairman of the Department of Orthopedic Surgery at Boston University, says, "The best types of exercise are those in which the pattern of effort or energy expenditure is continuous, such as jogging, swimming, or bicycling." He adds that singles tennis (not doubles) and fast walking are also good. He agrees that "many people, particularly those who have been basically inactive for a long time, require an element of social interaction in their exercise. . . . Some people also need some competition to keep them interested in physical activity and find running, swimming, and cycling boring and tedious—too much like work."

You have to pick the activity that best suits your personality and lifestyle and that can be done in your area's climate. If your spouse or lover agrees to leave your warm bed at the crack of dawn and hit the pavement with you, chatting as you walk, run, or cycle, then that is your choice. Or you may prefer a group of sweating, dancing bodies after work. If you are a solitary type who likes to suffer alone at sunup, or who loves the water because chatter is shielded from your ears, run off or dive off by yourself. There are no rules about whether you should exercise alone or in a group. It's up to you.

If you decide to jog, measure off a one-mile course in an out-of-the-way location not too far from where you live. If it has a soft, level surface, all the better, although you may have to resolve to run on pavement.

Buy yourself the best pair of running shoes you can afford. Uppers should be soft and nonirritating, toe room should be adequate, and heels should be half an inch higher than toes and protected. Sole material should be durable.

Dress lightly for the warm weather. Forget expensive jogging suits and rubberized clothes sold with the promise of your losing extra weight. All you will lose will be sweat.

Warm up with a few stretching exercises, then try your first mile. Accept the fact that you probably won't be able to run it. Don't be discouraged about having to walk most of your first mile after jogging a bit.

Run three times a week, and don't try to break any speed records. After a few weeks you'll be jogging a mile in 10 to 15 minutes. You should work up to 3 miles at a time for a 45-minute run that will burn off 450 extra calories.

Because bicycling is also a land-propulsion activity, it has the same shortcoming as jogging—an overdevelopment of certain leg muscles to the exclusion of others, and of other parts of your body. You need a safe road free of traffic lights and a good, light bike. A 150-pound cyclist burns an extra 255 calories per hour.

The best all-around exercise is swimming. If you can swim a mile, or even a half-mile, at a reasonable rate, just about all your skeletal muscles, plus your heart and lungs, will get decent workouts. Also, swimming is less punishing to feet, knees, and back than jogging is. And swimming is social. You get to meet people dressed only in bathing suits at poolside.

But swimming takes patience. You already know how to walk and run. You may have to learn how to swim. Even if you know how, you should learn the newest and most efficient versions of the four basic strokes: crawl, or free-style; backstroke; breast stroke; and butterfly.

Finally, you need a body of water. Large indoor "olympic-sized" (25 yards or longer) pools are best. Try to pick a time when the water is not churning with kids and then you won't be interrupted from swimming continuously.

Lakes or oceans are excellent in summer—if you can find a stretch that is patroled. Or an outdoor pool. Never, but never, swim alone.

Start out slowly, perhaps at first swimming a few lengths of the pool by sidestroke. Build yourself up to 5 and 10 lengths. Try the crawl and the other strokes. Do a quarter of a mile, then half a mile, three quarters and, finally, a mile.

Once you get in shape, you will find that you are converted to your regular exercise. You will be converted in the sense of being religious about it. Skip your regular run or swim or cycle, and you'll feel guilty. But after a workout, you will feel the warm glow of righteousness. With it goes trimness. And godliness.

How about the Sabbath Swim?

June — Week 2

With June busting out all over, fresh, locally grown fruit is appearing on roadside stands and in supermarkets. But before you scoop up too many berries, drown them in cream, and cover them with brown sugar, you'd better have some idea of the load of calories you'll be eating. Fruit is great food, but most kinds are loaded with their own sugar, so if you gorge on fruit, you'll likely find yourself busting out all over too.

Food	Calories
Cottage cheese	260
Watermelon	110
Cantaloupe	80
Honeydew	50
Orange	35
Grapefruit	25
Pineapple	40
Cherries, grapes, or blueberries	45
Bread	70
Butter or margarine	35
Wine	85
Sour cream	25
Total	860

For instance, a typical fruit plate is a mound of cottage cheese surrounded by an assortment of juicy hunks of fresh fruit, over which are sprinkled cherries, grapes, or blueberries. Side dishes offer sour cream, a slice of bread, and a pat of butter or margarine. A glass of cool, white dry wine may be at hand. The chart above shows the calorie count.

As you can see, this is not exactly low-cal.

Here's a more complete list of fruits and their calories. You should be able to integrate these amounts into your diet with little trouble. Watch out for the accompaniments, in which caloric danger lurks.

Fruit	Calories
Apple, raw, whole, 1 small (2-inch diameter)	58
Avocado, raw, peeled and pitted, ½ (3¼ by 4 inches)	167
Blackberries, raw, 1 cup	84
Blueberries, raw, 1 cup	87
Cantaloupe, raw, ¼ melon (5-inch diameter)	30
Cherries, sweet, raw, 15 large or 25 small	70
Fruit cocktail, water-packed, ½ cup scant	37
Grapes, American, 22 medium	69
Grapefruit, half	41
Honeydew melon, raw, ¼ small (5-inch diameter)	33
Loganberries, raw, ⅔ cup	62
Oranges, whole, 1 small (2½-inch diameter)	49
Peaches, raw, 1 medium	38
Pears, raw, ½ pear (3 by 2½ inches)	61
Pineapple, raw, diced, ¾ cup	52
Plums, damson, raw, 2 medium	66
Raisins, seedless, 1 tablespoon	29
Raspberries, black, raw, ⅔ cup	73
Raspberries, red, raw, ¾ cup	57
Strawberries, raw, 10 large	37
Watermelon, balls or cubes, 1¼ cup	26
Accompaniments	
Cottage cheese, 1 rounded teaspoon	30
Yogurt or skim milk, 1 cup	122
Sour cream, 1 ounce	57
Cream (half-and-half), 1 ounce	40
Brown sugar, 1 tablespoon	52
White sugar, 1 rounded teaspoon	32
Butterscotch sauce, 2 tablespoons	203
Chocolate sauce, 2 tablespoons	87
Custard sauce, ¼ cup	85
Hollandaise sauce, ¼ cup	180
Lemon sauce, ¼ cup	133
Sour cream sauce, ¼ cup	141

June — Week 3

Wives need to know how best to help their husbands lose weight. So, for Father's Day, here are a dozen rules for wives of dieting husbands.

1. *Support him every chance you get.* He cannot do it alone. He needs your help.

2. *Don't nag.* Gently make him aware of it when he slips into his old eating habits. Breaking old habits is very difficult; reverting to them is very easy. Don't remind him in public, but do let him know, quietly, when he behaves with food as he doesn't want to.

3. *Be neither mother nor police officer.* Instead, be a social worker. Offer to work out his problems with him. Dieting will impose an extra stress on your relationship. There are enough outside pressures pulling married couples apart these days, and you don't need to worsen things by intensifying internal pressures.

4. *Be sensitive.* When his nervous nibbling returns—and it will—that's a clue that something may be upsetting him. When you two are alone and you have the opportunity, tell him that you notice he is troubled and offer to let him talk it out with you.

5. *Don't express your love with food.* Don't ever push seconds at him. Use other physical expressions, such as touching, kissing, embracing. When grocery shopping, and you want to buy something to delight him, don't pick a gooey cake off the shelf or a new ice cream flavor from the freezer. Instead, find him something with few if any calories, such as a special tea or an exotic vegetable or fruit. Or a humorous greeting card.

6. *Don't use food as a reward.* He doesn't "deserve" a half-gallon of ice cream after jogging or swimming or working out in the gym. As a matter of fact, strenuous exercise curbs the appetite. You should reinforce this feeling. Moreover, increased physical activity and decreased calories work well together to burn off fat.

7. *Ask him to help plan the meals you eat together.* Sit down together and make up your shopping lists. Buy only as much food as necessary, no more. If you buy too much, you'll find you are pushing the food on him because "it's a sin to throw it out."

8. *Eat what he eats.* Don't let him feel like a freak, eating his "diet food" while you and the kids eat something else. The social aspects should be the focus of family dinners, not the food.

9. *Don't buy noshes and nibbles and leave them around the house.* The temptation to nibble is never so strong as when someone else offers the food. In a way, this gives him permission to overeat even though he knows better.

10. *Tell him he looks nice.* And back up your compliments once in a while by buying him a present of some new clothes. Buy a standard size picked off a rack, rather than from a fat man's haberdashery. Never cut him down with remarks like "You really are getting too skinny." Be happy he thinks enough of himself to want to be thin. If he is to love you, and return your love, he must like himself first.

11. *Don't compete with his fitness program.* You should not regard the time he spends exercising as time stolen from you. It's his personal time. And this is time invested in your future because he'll probably live longer if he's fit.

12. *Don't be jealous of his new slimness.* If you have to lose weight, too, do it. If you can't, don't blame him for your failure.

June — Week 4

In preparation for America's birthday, you can be on the Great American Diet. (This is not to be confused with the 1982 book, *The I Love America Diet.*)

It's cheap. You can obtain a copy from the U.S. Government Printing Office, Washington, DC 20402. Ask for *Dietary Goals for the United States,* second edition (1977). A condensed version, *Nutrition and Your Health,* is also available from the U.S. GPO. Ask for Home and Garden Bulletin No. 232.

It's safe. These publications spell out a diet you can live on for the rest of your life. And if you live on this diet, your life may be longer than it would have been on your unhealthy diet. With this diet you'll lose weight, keep it off, and have healthier arteries, veins, heart, and digestive system.

It has integrity. Unlike any fad diet you've heard about or followed, it does not have as its major ingredient baloney.

It's controversial. This government diet has been under attack by the meat industry, the dairy industry, and segments of the medical establishment. But the American Heart Association and leading nutritionists think it's the greatest.

The major points raised by the objectors are that the government diet would severely change food purchasing patterns in the marketplace and that it would represent a major shift in American eating practices.

But that is what the book is all about. It is a distillation of the recommendations of top food and health experts in the United States and abroad, who provided written and oral testimony to Senator George McGovern and his Select Committee on Nutrition and Human Needs.

The report addresses overweight early on. "Obesity resulting from the over-consumption of calories is a major risk factor in killer diseases. Therefore, it is extremely important either to maintain an optimal weight, or to alter one's weight to reach an optimal level.

"Obesity is associated with the onset and clinical progression of diseases such as

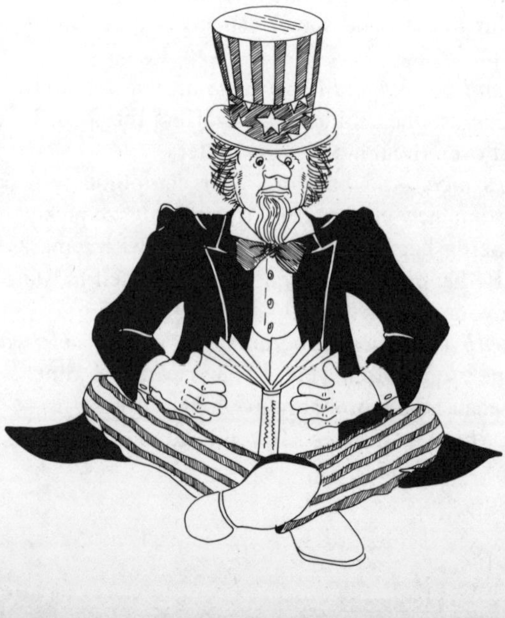

hypertension, diabetes mellitus, heart disease and gall bladder disease. It may also modify the quality of one's life."

In addition to losing weight and keeping it off, the report lists six other dietary goals:

1. Increase the consumption of complex carbohydrates (starches) and "naturally occurring sugars" (in fruits), from 28 percent of daily total calories to 48 percent.
2. At the same time, halve the amount of refined sugar we eat every day, from 18 percent of daily calories to 10 percent.
3. Eat less fat (from 40 percent of daily calories to 30 percent).
4. Balance the kinds of fats we eat so that 10 percent of daily calories are saturated fats (like butter, which are firm at room temperature) and 10 percent are polyunsaturated fats (runny oils such as safflower and corn).
5. Hold daily cholesterol consumption to 300 milligrams a day (slightly less than the total amount of one egg yolk).
6. Eat no more than 5 grams of table salt a day.

To achieve these goals, the report recommends that you eat more fruits, vegetables, and whole grains and less refined sugar and high-fat foods (especially meat, eggs, butter, ice cream and other high-milk-fat dairy foods). Replace whole milk with skim or low-fat milk.

This also means shifting from potato chips to baked potatoes, from canned fruit and vegetables to fresh ones, from white bread to whole wheat bread, from instant white rice to brown rice, and from sugar-coated breakfast cereals to plain cereals.

The recommended diet calls for the same 12 percent protein content as before, but for increased amounts of carbohydrates (from 46 to 58 percent), with decreased amounts of fats (from 42 percent to 30 percent).

In practical terms, this means that on a daily 1,200-calorie reducing diet, you would be eating 144 calories of protein, 696 calories of carbohydrate, and 360 calories of fat. By quantity, this is 36 grams of protein, 174 grams of carbohydrate, and 40 grams of fat.

Maybe you immediately see the problem here: not enough protein. As an adult, you need half again as much: about 60 grams. This means the calculations are OK for a 2,000-calorie maintenance diet. But on a diet to lose weight, with restricted calories, you need to eat more protein than 12 percent of total calories.

The solution is easy: Replace some of the carbohydrates with protein. To do this without raising fat calories, replace meat with high-protein legumes (beans).

When doing your arithmetic, remember that proteins and carbohydrates are 4 calories per gram; fat is 9 calories per gram. Treat alcoholic beverages like carbohydrates; alcohol is 7 calories per gram.

There it is. It may not be easy, but it is the best around. The little work and preparation required are offset by the benefits, which are long range and well worth it.

Of course, if you have trouble with arithmetic, there is yet another publication to help you. It is *Food-2*, published by the American Dietetic Association, Dept. DA, 430 North Michigan Avenue, Chicago, IL 60611. *Food-2* offers 1,200-, 1,500-, and 1,800-calorie daily menus plus 22 pages of recipes, all based on dietary goals and each identified by total calories, total fat, saturated fat, and cholesterol per serving. You can get *Food-2* and *Food-3*, a companion volume, from the ADA for $7.50 plus a $2.00 shipping charge.

Whichever publication you choose, do it. Give yourself an American birthday present for life.

THE GREAT AMERICAN DIET (1800 CALORIES)

BREAKFAST
Orange juice, ¾ cup
Poached egg, 1
Bran muffins, 2
Margarine, 2 teaspoons
Skim milk, 1 cup

LUNCH
Split pea soup, 1 cup
Chicken salad sandwich
Chicken salad, ½ cup made with low-calorie mayonnaise-type salad dressing
rye bread, 2 slices
Pear, canned in light syrup, 2 small halves with syrup
Water, tea, or coffee

DINNER
Sweet and sour pork chops, 1 serving
Baked sweet potato, 1 small
Broccoli, cooked, ½ cup
Fruit cup, ⅔ cup (apples, oranges, bananas)
Whole wheat roll, 1
Margarine, 1 teaspoon
Water tea, or coffee

SNACK
Skim milk, 1 cup
Whole wheat crackers, 4

(1500 CALORIES)

BREAKFAST
Grapefruit juice unsweetened, ½ cup
Shredded wheat, 1 biscuit
Whole wheat toast, 1 slice
Margarine, 1 teaspoon
Skim milk, ½ cup

LUNCH
Roast beef sandwich
Roast beef, cooked, lean, 3 ounces
Lettuce leaf,1
Mayonnaise-type salad dressing, 2 teaspoons
Whole wheat bread, 2 slices
Carrot strips, 6 to 8 (2½ - 3 inches long)
Orange, 1 medium
Water, tea, or coffee

DINNER
Baked fish fillet, 1 serving
Baked potato, 1
Margarine, 2 teaspoons
Green peas, cooked, ½ cup
Salad
Tomato, sliced ½
Cucumber, sliced ½
Yogurt-dill dressing, 2 tablespoons
French bread, 1 medium slice
Margarine, 1 teaspoon
Peach slices, fresh, ½ cup
Water, tea, or coffee

SNACK
Plain low-fat yogurt, ¾ cup with blueberries fresh or frozen (unsweetened), ¼ cup

(1200 CALORIES)

BREAKFAST
Bran flakes, ¾ cup with strawberries, fresh, ¾ cup and plain low-fat yogurt, ¾ cup

LUNCH
Chef's salad, 1 serving
Salad dressing, Italian, regular, 2 tablespoons
Rye wafers, 4
Tangerine, 1 medium
Water, tea, or coffee.

DINNER
Mock Beef Stroganoff (with noodles), 1 serving
Spinach, cooked, ½ cup
Whole wheat roll, 1
Margarine, 1 teaspoon
Cantaloupe, 5-inch diameter, ¼
Skim milk, 1 cup

SNACK
Banana, 1 medium

July — Week 1

In honor of the Fourth of July, let's look at a fat Founding Father.

Although he practiced moderation during his lean days in the colonies, Benjamin Franklin's diet was carbohydrate heavy. His calories and weight increased when he went to France, where sauces, desserts, and wine were served as a matter of protocol.

Franklin's advice is applicable today: "Those who move much may, and indeed ought to, eat more; those who use little exercise should eat little. In general, mankind since the improvement of cookery eats about twice as much as nature requires."

Franklin became a vegetarian when he was 16. A colonial staple, hasty pudding, worked well in this meatless diet. A mush made of cornmeal, egg yolk, milk, and bread crumbs, it often was served for dinner. Leftovers were fried in butter or bacon fat for breakfast. But at the age of 17, on a boat to New York, Franklin went back to eating cod, and returned "only now and then to a vegetable diet."

Franklin loved carbohydrates. In October 1723, on his first day in Philadelphia, he "walked toward the top of the street, gazing about till near Market Street, when I met a boy with bread. I had often made a meal of dry bread, and inquiring where he had bought it, I went immediately to the baker's he directed me to. I asked for biscuits, meaning such as we had at Boston; that sort, it seems, was not made at Philadelphia. I then asked for a threepenny loaf and was told they had none. Not knowing the different prices nor the names of the different sorts of bread, I told him to give me threepenny worth of any sort. He gave me accordingly three great puffy rolls. I was surprised at the quantity but took it and, having no room in my pockets, walked off with a roll under each arm and eating the other.

"Thus I went up Market Street as far as Fourth Street, passing by the door of Mr. Read, my future wife's father; when she, standing at the door, saw me, and thought I made, as certainly I did, a most awkward, ridiculous appearance. Then I turned and went down Chestnut Street and part of Walnut Street, eating my roll all the way; and coming round found myself again at Market Street wharf, near the boat I came in, to which I went for a draught of river water; and being filled with one of my rolls, gave the other two to a woman and her child."

In relating how moderate he was, Franklin explained, "My breakfast for a long time was bread and milk (no tea), and I eat it out of twopenny earthen porringer with a pewter spoon."

Franklin went to work for a fat printer named Keimer, with whom he later roomed. He tried to get Keimer to lose weight:

"Our provisions were purchased, cooked, and brought to us regularly by a woman in the neighborhood, who had from me a list of 40 dishes which she prepared for us at different times, in which there entered neither fish, flesh, nor fowl.

"I went on pleasantly, but poor Keimer suffered grievously, grew tired of the project, longed for the fleshpots of Egypt, and ordered a roast pig. He invited me and two women friends to dine with him, but, it being brought too soon upon table, he could not resist the temptation and ate the whole before we came."

Keimer had violated Franklin's first moral virtue: "Temperance—eat not to dullness; drink not to elevation."

That Franklin followed Poor Richard's advice for most of his life—"Eat to live, and not live to eat"—may have been a factor in his longevity. He died at age 84 in 1790.

July — Week 2

Take this book along with you on your travels. For this week features a guide to dieting while on an auto trip.

Driving for long hours can be boring, offering the temptation to nibble. You should anticipate nibbling in advance by bringing along a bag of hard diet candies made with sugar substitutes and virtually calorie free. (Shun any so-called diet chocolate.)

Also bring along a thermos of coffee, tea, or cold water and pour a cup whenever you feel thirsty or drowsy on the road. Since coffee and tea contain caffeine, a diuretic, you will have to make stops every couple of hours. *Caution:* Don't fill up your tummy while filling your car's gas tank. Stay away from the candy machine and the ice cream counter.

Keep your hands busy when you are not driving. Macrame—the craft of knotting—is good. So is needlework. Catch up on reading and letter writing. All these activities should keep your mind off food.

When you stop for a meal, the temptations you find may be overwhelming. Merely getting to the roadside restaurant or cafeteria is dangerous. You walk through Candy Land, with caramel popcorn, pecan rolls, oversize lollipops, and other sweets beckoning to you from racks and counters.

For dieters, the only good thing about food along the road is its high price, which may deter you. But in the unreal and unrestrained world of the open road, you may suddenly feel like ordering a chocolate soda and some clam chowder for lunch, and may even want them served in that order. Or you may, if you are in a hurry, walk off with a hamburger, fries, and a shake from the carry-out counter and gobble them down before you reach the car.

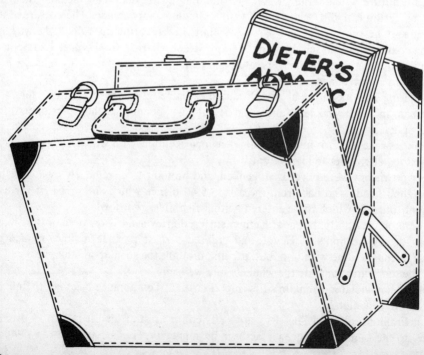

Your first food stop is very important. It will set the tone of your meals on the entire trip. So sit down and eat your meal. Don't grab foods and wolf them down while standing. Order only food that is on your diet plan, whether it be salad or broiled fish. Don't select everything that tempts you on the cafeteria serving line. Don't eat off the plates of your spouse and children. If you ask for saccharine or another sugar substitute in most restaurants or cafeterias, you will get it. Similarly, you don't have to take the cream that is usually served with cereal for breakfast; ask for skim milk instead. Never be bashful or embarrassed about your dieting or its requirements.

An even better idea on the road is to avoid restaurants, cafeterias, and carry-out counters and picnic instead. This mobile method of brown bagging ensures your planning meals rationally and in advance. There are other advantages: It's cheaper, you don't have to wait to be served, and you can spend some time out-of-doors enjoying the forests, mountains, or other scenery you would otherwise zip past. There is nothing quite as refreshing as resting by a cool mountain stream. The peace will ease your nerves and calm your spirit.

After you check into the motel and your family settles down for the night, you'll have the usual bored-evening "munchies," highlighted by the letdown of tension away from the wheel. Although your kitchen refrigerator is not at hand, there are Coke and candy dispensers down the corridor.

Prepare for these nights by bringing along instant coffee or tea bags and a plug-in water boiler. Or, if you like iced tea, bring instant tea and send one of your kids to get ice from the machine down the hall.

Many soda pop dispensers in motels offer diet drinks. But if you don't want to pay the outrageous price and want to be sure you get your favorite brand and flavor, buy your own six-pack.

One last tip: Try eating only two meals. If you leave the motel at 6 A.M., you can survive with your thermos of coffee and drive until 10, then pull off for brunch. Pull off again at 2 P.M. and have cold noncaloric drinks. You stop and check in at 6, eat dinner at 7, and have hot coffee in the room at 10 P.M. If you take your children, let them nibble cold cereal early in the morning in the back of the car.

As for exercise, try jogging around every gas station at which you stop; and pick motels that have pools. Nothing is as relaxing and refreshing as a swim at the end of a hard day's drive.

July — Week 3

Dieters who exercise in hot weather need to be very careful. Otherwise, heat cramps, heat exhaustion, or even heat stroke can strike.

These often are delayed reactions. Marathon runner Bob Glover recalled, "I ran 20 miles in warm humid weather, then took a quick shower and went off to the lecture without eating or replacing fluids. The room was warm and stuffy and held more than 400 people, mostly doctors, who listened intently as I delivered my slide presentation. Suddenly, I was having trouble remembering my carefully written speech; I began asking the slide projectionist to please focus the slides. The next thing I knew I was on the floor."

Glover quickly recovered with water and cooling. But he learned a lesson: Heat puts a severe stress on the body.

Glover, in his *Runner's Handbook* (Penguin, 1978) advises that in hot weather you need to take periodic rest breaks; dress carefully—white and lightweight clothes, preferably cotton; drink plenty of liquids before, during, and after running; keep your body

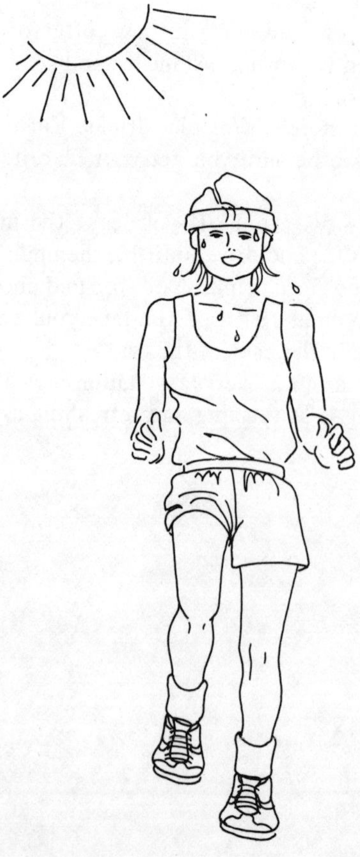

wet, either with your own sweat or with water poured over your head; run on cool surfaces, choosing grass instead of pavement, or the beach at the water line.

The Running Book (Consumer Guide, 1978) suggests that you not run when the thermometer exceeds 85 degrees F, particularly when it's humid, and especially if you are overweight and over age 40. And if the sun is out, wear a hat.

The body requires about two weeks to acclimatize to warm weather. Unfortunately, bodies that live in air-conditioned comfort don't get this chance. That is one reason you have to be especially careful when jogging, playing tennis or racquetball, or participating in any strenuous activity in the heat.

As a dieter, you are constantly concerned with heat, whether you know it or not. The calorie is a measure of heat generated as your body uses energy. You know this energy comes in food: Eat more than you burn and you accumulate fat; eat less, and you lose fat.

Dr. Joseph M. Quashnock, commander of the Air Force's School of Aerospace Medicine, says, "The human body is a heat-producing engine that must maintain its temperature within rather narrow limits." In summer your body, like your car, is fighting outside heat as it tries to maintain its internal temperature. In health, your body temperature varies no more than one degree from 98.6 degrees F.

You know that when you use your muscles, you burn calories. Another way of saying this is that when your muscles work, they generate heat. At rest, your muscles contribute only about a quarter of your body's heat. Exercise moderately, and this amount doubles. Exercise strenuously, and their heat production can soar to 2,000 percent.

At rest, you lose about an ounce of water an hour as perspiration. As sweat evaporates, it cools. If the air around you is dry, it soaks up the sweat, and you feel cool. But if the air is muggy, the sweat sits there, and you feel dripping wet and no cooler. Under such conditions, you may sweat heavily—and may lose up to 3.5 quarts of water an hour. The weight you lose is all water.

If you read labels, you know that water is a major ingredient of most foods. So if you are limiting the amount of food you eat, you are also limiting the amount of water you are getting.

When you sweat heavily, other things happen. Your kidneys conserve water and, as a consequence, secrete a concentrated, dark urine that is loaded with potassium. As body tissues lose water, some cells die. As it sweats, your body gives up sodium.

If your body cannot cool off, and its temperature goes up, you may feel dizzy or lightheaded and start breathing heavily. If your skin is pale and feels clammy, you are suffering heat exhaustion. When that happens, stop and sit down before you pass out. Get in the shade or other cool place or under a cool shower. Drink. Drink. Drink.

But if you drink only water, you may suffer heat cramps. This is, in effect, water intoxication, according to Dr. Quashnock. It is a sign that you need salt. A few pinches of salt in a glass of water should do it. Or drink tomato juice. But go easy on the salt when your stomach is empty.

Without taking any of these measures, you could go on to heat stroke, which is an acute and dangerous condition. It can damage the brain and even kill. Warning signs are headache, mental confusion, numbness and tingling, convulsions, and coma. Body temperature may be as high as 104 degrees F. If this happens to a buddy, pour on cold water and rub fingers and toes.

Better yet, your buddy and you should drink plenty of fruit juices, dress right, and pay attention to the thermometer so as to prevent heat complications.

July — Week 4

The nice part of camping and boating is that these out-of-door activities get you far away from the refrigerator and cookie jar. Still, out in the woods and on the water can lurk serious and hidden dangers for dieters. Unless you are prepared for them, you may easily succumb.

A major danger is the attitude that because you are drinking in that wonderful outdoor air and burning all those outdoor calories, you *deserve* to eat more. Sorry, but the fact is that pitching a tent, running a boat, and fishing burn up very few calories.

Yes, chopping down trees, hiking, or pedaling a bike for many miles will consume lots of extra calories. At the same time, the extra physical activity will curb your appetite. Instead of using the exercise as an excuse to consume marshmallows and other goodies around the fire, use it as a means of multiplying your weight loss as you diet.

The secret of dieting at camp or on a boat is planning. You need to plan every meal away from home. Shop according to the limitations of the barbecue grill and alcohol stove (and *never* shop on an empty stomach). Of course, you may get lucky and reel in some pan fish from that stream or lake. There are few finer gourmet delights, unmatched even by the fanciest four-star restaurants, than a fish cooked fresh from the water. It depends on the type of fish, but grilling is better (in terms of fewer calories) than frying. If fry you must, use a Teflon-lined pan which requires no fat. Since fish is probably a staple on your diet, take along some cans of water-packed tuna, crab, and salmon, and some cans of sardines, just in case the live ones aren't biting. (If they are, you can always bring the cans home.)

Also, take along yogurt and cottage cheese. Both keep well in a cooler or icebox and can be served at breakfast or lunch. A cup of plain yogurt is only 125 calories; a cup of uncreamed cottage cheese is only 170 calories.

Take along lots of the lower-calorie fresh fruit available now, especially grapes, peaches, plums, and nectarines, as well as oranges, grapefruit, and apples. If you have room, take cantaloupe too. Carrots, celery, and cauliflower keep well in coolers and provide between-meal nibbles. Take plenty of instant coffee, tea, and diet soda.

Fortunately, ice cream doesn't keep in a cooler, so you can't take any along. Neither should you bring cookies, sweet rolls, cake, or sugar candy. And no bread. Crackers or matzos keep better and offer fewer calories.

If you hike or cycle, you can't pack as much, so you may prefer freeze-dried foods. Stay away from those with cream sauce or heavy gravy. But don't forsake the old camping standby, pork and beans. In a one-cup can are 16 grams of protein. Add a slice of rye bread, and you have a 370-calorie dinner.

Freeze-dried vegetables are especially good. If your camping or boating situation allows for the use of a wok, you can bring it to make stir-fried Asian dishes that are heavy on vegetables.

Some camp-out dieters find that they do best by prepackaging their own meals, especially dinners. They slice the meat and cheese and prepare the low-calorie sauces they'll use while away, then wrap them in aluminum and plastic for the cooler. Besides controlling calories, this technique also shortens meal preparation and allows you more time to marvel at the sight and silence of nature.

An unseen danger outdoors is the mixture that goes under various names, including Trail Mix and California Mix. This may well serve skinny college kids on mountain hikes, but the mixes are too loaded with calories (mainly in the oils of the seeds and nuts) for the rest of us. And don't fall for the pitch about carob being a great diet substitute for chocolate. You save only a few calories. Better stay away from both.

If you are a Trail Mix addict, mix up your own. The bulk should come from a dry cereal such as Cracklin' Bran and not one of the sugar-coated ones or a commercial granola. A handful of dry cereal contains far fewer calories than a handful of nuts (50 versus 200 calories). For flavor, sparingly add sunflower seeds (half a cup is 400 calories), shredded coconut (half a cup is 150 calories), raisins (half a cup is 210 calories), prunes (half a cup is 250 calories), dried apricot (half a cup is 170 calories), and almonds (half a cup is 400 calories).

Finally, a bit of philosophy. Time was, many millennia ago, when your forebears knew how to live off the land. They were skilled at catching fish, trapping small animals, and hunting big animals, all for food. They knew how to sow and harvest crops. Many generations later, you are a civilized descendant. You express a contempt of civilization by getting out-of-doors now and then. Still, you have to take your necessities with you. You have to carry along your home comforts, somewhat as a turtle carries its home along.

You are very susceptible to Civilized Panic when you fear that out in the forest you will not have enough to eat. That's understandable; eating is basic to survival. But the fear is not subject to reason; it is purely emotional. It is the feeling that you cannot survive, as your forebears did, off the land.

The most obvious manifestation of this fear is overbuying and overpacking vittles (as the pioneers used to call their food). But that isn't the end of it. Inside your head, you have this recorded message that keeps telling you that it is a sin to waste food, that there are millions of people starving around the world, and that what you throw out would feed them for a week. So your appetite expands to consume all the food you have brought along, even though you know you brought too much.

It's hard to conquer primeval fears of starvation in the wilderness. But remember that even in the most remote areas of the Rockies and Alaska, you can get to a store or a restaurant before you starve. So, as a rule, halve the amount of food you plan to bring on the boat or to camp.

And have a good time. The peacefulness of the outdoors will do wonders to calm your nerves, perhaps even to the point of removing, at least temporarily, the anxiety that causes you to nibble and overeat.

July — Week 5

You'd think that with life so casual during the summer, dieting would be easier. It isn't. In fact, this is probably the hardest time of the year to try to lose weight. Blame the thirst quenchers; the junk you eat at the ball game, picnic, beach, or amusement park; and those patio parties.

To sensitize you to summer seductions of the palate, here is a discussion and some data.

Many dieters in summer turn to salads for lunch: fruit and cottage cheese (860 calories), crab Louis (875), and julienne (970).

Sandwiches usually are lower in calories: Big Mac (561), hot dog with trimmings (250), grilled cheese (250), corned beef on rye (450). Even a wedge of Pizza Hut Supreme is lower (475). But who can eat only one?

Summer also offers many opportunities—and excuses—to overeat. You are out

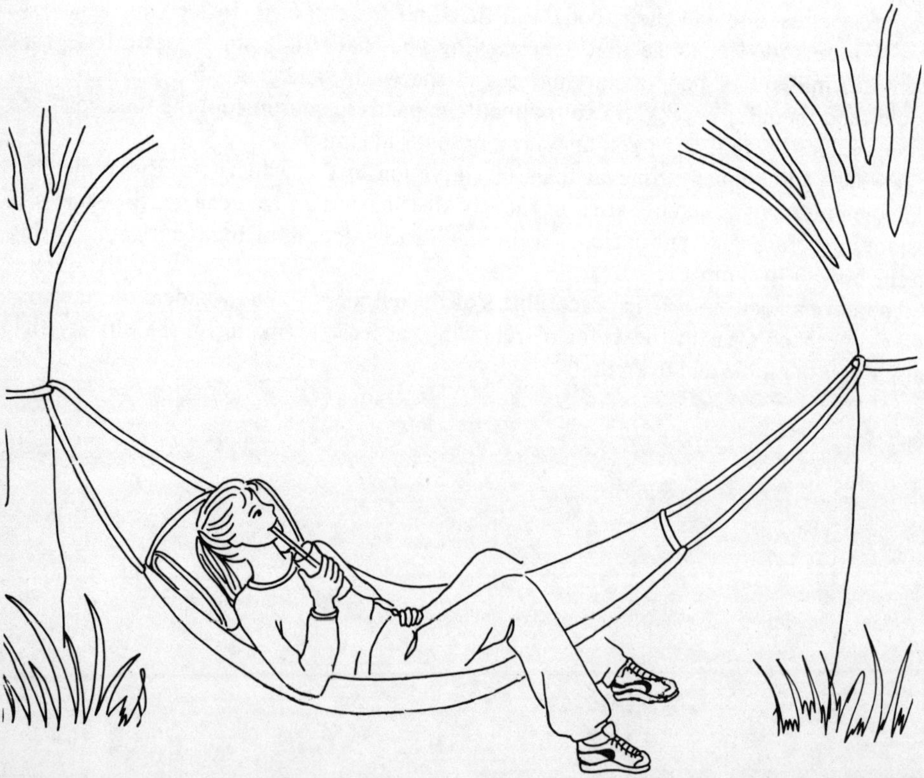

more, among people more. And it's hard to resist an offer of something cold to drink when you're hot and sweaty.

One of the oldest favorites is lemonade, sold on the streets by children and easy to make from powder mixes or frozen concentrate. Each cold, refreshing glass will contribute 103 calories and not much else. Lemonade is essentially sugar and water and lemon flavor with a bit of vitamin C.

Orangeade is not much better. The ingredients of a popular orangeade mix are sugar, citric acid (provides tartness), imitation and natural flavors, cellulose gum (adds body), salt, dextrin, ascorbic acid (vitamin C), U.S.-certified artificial colors, vegetable shortening, and dehydrated orange juice. The label adds that the orangeade "contains less than 5 percent orange juice" and that a glass gives you 90 calories, 22 grams of carbohydrate, 10 percent of your daily allowance of vitamin C, and no protein or fat.

Nutional information is listed on the package or bottle or cap because the law requires it. Nutritional labeling is one of the best things to happen to dieters in years. The ingredients are listed by rank, with the major ingredients first, the least last.

Here are the ingredients listed for another popular cold drink, cola: carbonated water, sugar, caramel color, phosphoric acid, natural flavorings, caffeine. A 12-ounce can gives you 145 calories as sugar dissolved in colored fizz water. The uncola soft drink is not much better.

Ice-cold beer is another favorite summer thirst quencher. The contents of each 12-ounce can total 150 calories.

The accompanying chart shows how other summer coolers with alcohol rate calorically:

Drink	**Calories**
Bloody Mary	217
Cuba libre	211
Daiquiri	167
Gimlet	148
Gin and tonic	175
Grasshopper	272
Highball	166
Manhattan	164
Margarita	146
Mint julep	212
Old fashioned	179
Planter's punch	175
Rum collins	207
Screwdriver	227
Tom collins	217
Whiskey sour	163
Wine, white	85
Zombie	549

Not everyone quenches thirst with alcoholic beverages. Many forgo alcohol for ice cream, claiming there is nothing as throat soothing as a chocolate ice cream soda, shake, or malted (255, 421, and 502 calories respectively).

Also, an ice cream bar has 180 calories; an ice cream sandwich, 173, and an ice cream cone (2 scoops), 400.

Watermelon is 115 calories for an 8-inch by 4-inch wedge.

There is nothing better for quenching thirst than plain tap water and ice. No calories, period. And no expense. Or if it is very warm, try some plain seltzer, fizz water, or club soda on ice. If you want taste, then drink artificially sweetened soda pop. But watch your quantity. Saccharine is safe in small quantities, but it *is* artificial.

If you haven't tried iced tea or iced coffee, you are in for a surprise. A cup of tea contains 2 calories, and a cup of black coffee contains 35 calories. On the rocks with a little bit of saccharine, either drink is low in calories, low in cost, and very high in thirst-satisfying effectiveness. Add a cinnamon stick for novelty.

August — Week 1

This is a good season to get lots of fiber into your diet. And if you do, you will accelerate your weight loss. That's because, explains Audrey Eaton, fiber "steals" calories from the food you eat. In her book, *The F-Plan Diet* (Crown, 1983), she says, "When people eat high-fiber diets they excrete more calories in their stools[feces]. . . nearly 10 percent."

Fiber is the stuff in food that cows and other ruminants can digest, but people cannot. It is only in plants and never in food derived from animals. Fiber is mainly cellulose, with a few other components. It is not to be confused with "fibrous," which describes the texture of some meats.

The slimming benefits of fiber in your food "start in the mouth, continue in the stomach, extend to the blood, and reach a grand finale with that final flush!" Eaton writes.

Eaton's enthusiasm for what occurs in the bowels is not scatological. That's where the action is. The fiber—it used to be called roughage—increases the bulk in your intestines and stimulates them to move things along at a quicker pace than otherwise. The speed is great enough to somewhat foil the efforts of the walls of the intestines to extract every last nutrient from the digested food. This, according to the research Eaton quoted, accounts for the 10 percent shortfall in calories.

Eaton's diet followed by a decade research by Dr. Denis Burkitt, the Irish surgeon who put "fiber" in everyday conversation. He brought about an appreciation of fiber in the 1970s that was, in fact, a scientific renaissance of the value of "roughage" promoted by cereal-makers Kellogg and Post in the 1890s.

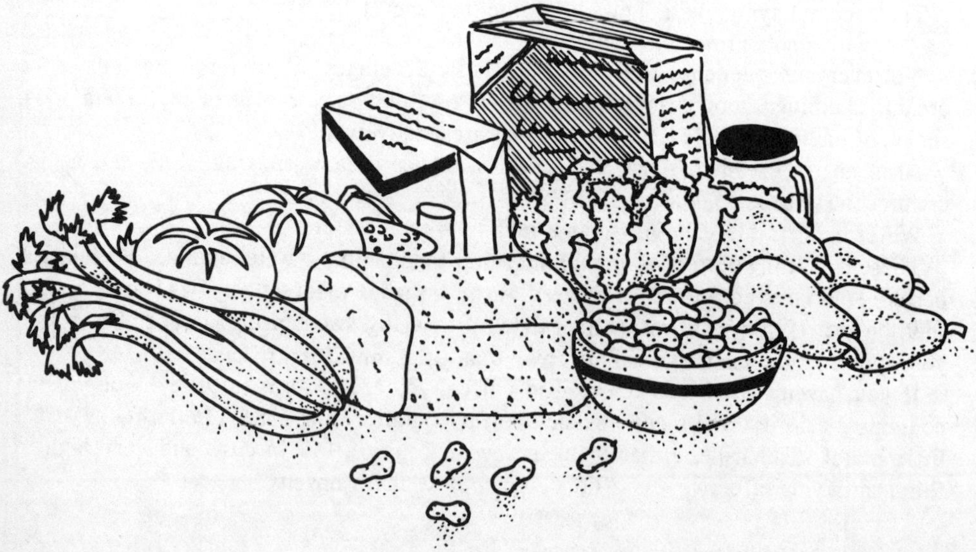

Dr. Burkitt studied the stools of English and African natives and concluded that the amount of dietary fiber was the variable which accounted for a high incidence of bowel cancer in the former but a low incidence in the latter.

With little bulk in the diet, the English bowel held digested food for long periods of time. This was long enough to allow every nutritional iota to be absorbed and for the digested food to ferment and produce noxious chemicals that irritated the lining of the bowel. If chronic, it promoted the induction of cancer and other diseases. When the bowel finally did discharge its contents, they were small, hard, smelly, dry stools.

By contrast, the African's stool was large, soft, moist, and seldom smelled. This was because the digested food, heavy with fiber, absorbed lots of moisture and moved rapidly through the gut. There was no time for it to ferment, nor enough time to surrender every bit of nutrient.

This last phenomenon is what makes fiber a great diet gimmick. The Africans in the study were much slimmer than the Britons. In *Eat Right—To Stay Healthy and Enjoy Life More* (Arco, 1979), Dr. Burkitt explains: "Obesity occurs if energy[calories] *absorbed* from the food eaten exceeds the energy used in the functions of the body. High-fiber foods reduce not only the amount of energy consumed but also decrease absorption of energy."

Eaton found that fiber's advantages start with the process of eating. High-fiber foods such as apples, baked beans, and chickpeas act to slow down your eating because they have to be thoroughly chewed before they can be comfortably swallowed. This chewing satisfies most of your need to have food in your mouth.Thus, high-fiber foods obviate the need for much other food, especially high-calorie foods that you gulp down without paying much attention.

Once in your stomach, high-fiber foods absorb and hold water; they swell in your stomach to lend that filled-up feeling. Once the foods leave the stomach, their bulk moves them quickly along through the small and large intestines toward elimination.

Eaton suggests that you take between 35 and 50 grams of fiber daily. Because you may not be able to derive this much fiber from the foods you eat on a low-calorie diet, she devised a mixture called Fiber Filler, which yields 15 grams of fiber—more than most people consume a day. The ingredients:

⅓ cup, 40 Percent Bran Flakes
3 tablespoons bran meal
3 tablespoons Bran Buds or All-Bran
2 tablespoons sliced almonds
1 large prune, pitted and chopped
2 dried apricot halves, chopped
1 tablespoon raisins

Since this mixture totals 200 calories, you need to deduct that amount from your daily intake. You need to deduct yet another 200 calories for a cup of skim milk and two pieces of fruit, which Eaton advises you take with Fiber Filler. Total calories: 400. Total fiber: 20 grams.

You get the rest of the fiber in the foods you select for your other meals, from a handy list Eaton provides in her book. Incidentally, she credited this list to Dr. James W. Anderson of the Veterans Administration Medical Center, Lexington, Kentucky. Dr. Burkitt credited Dr. Anderson with having devised one of the best high-fiber weight-loss diets. (Two Lexington Diet days are reprinted in this chapter.)

There are other food fiber lists. Perhaps the most complete is *The Barbara Kraus Guide to Fiber in Foods* (Signet, 1975).

Another high-fiber diet that works is *Dr. Siegel's Natural Fiber Permanent Weight Loss Diet* (Dial Press, 1975). Also, just as a reminder, all vegetarian diets are high in fiber, emphasizing as they do fruits, vegetables, and whole-grain foods. So too are such modified vegetarian diets as *The Alternative Diet* (University of Iowa Publications, 1976) and *The Pritikin Permanent Weight-Loss Manual* (Bantam, 1981).

Eaton's top-20 fiber foods are

1. Dried beans, peas, and other legumes
2. Bran cereals
3. Lima beans
4. Green peas
5. Dried figs, apricots, and dates
6. Raspberries, blackberries, and strawberries
7. Sweet corn
8. Whole-wheat and other whole-grain cereal products
9. Broccoli
10. Potato
11. Beans: French, Italian, snap, pole, and broad
12. Apples, pears, and plums
13. Raisins and prunes
14. Greens: spinach, turnips, beets, kale, collards, and Swiss chard
15. Nuts
16. Cherries
17. Bananas
18. Carrots
19. Coconut
20. Brussels sprouts

KELLOGG'S 7-DAY FIBER DIET
(1200 Calories)

DAY 1

		Calories	Dietary Fiber in Grams
BREAKFAST			
½ cup	Grapefruit unsweetened	50	0
½ cup (1 oz.)	Kellogg's® Cracklin' Bran® cereal	110	4.0
1 slice	Whole wheat toast	50	2.1
1 pat	Butter (or margarine)	35	0
1 cup	Skim milk	85	0
1 cup	Coffee, black	5	0
		335	6.1
LUNCH			
	Ham and cheese sandwich:		
3 ounce	Ham, lean only	200	0
1 ounce	Swiss cheese	95	0
2 leaves	Lettuce	0	0.2
2 slices	Whole wheat bread	100	4.2
1 stalk	Celery	5	0.7
1 cup	Skim milk	85	0
		485	5.1
DINNER			
3 ounces	Fish fillet, flounder	120	0

1 tsp.	Lemon juice	0	0
½ cup	Carrots	15	2.3
½ cup	Asparagus, cut	15	1.1
½ slice	Bran banana bread	115	1.8
1 cup	Coffee, black	5	0
		270	5.2
SNACK			
1 medium	Apple, with peel	75	3.3
	Day's total	1165	19.7

DAY 2

BREAKFAST			
1 small	Orange	40	2.4
1 large	Egg, soft or hard cooked	80	0
2 slices	Cracked wheat toast	110	4.2
1 pat	Butter (or margarine)	35	0
1 cup	Skim milk	85	0
1 cup	Coffee, black	5	0
		355	6.8
LUNCH			
3 ounces	Fish sticks, breaded	205	0
1 tsp.	Tartar sauce	25	0
1	Carrot, raw	20	2.3
½ cup	Green beans	5	2.0
3	Rye wafers	65	2.3
1 cup	Skim milk	85	0
		405	6.6
DINNER			
3 ounces	Pork chop, lean (baked or roasted)	230	0
	Salad:		
1/6 head	Lettuce	10	1.4
1 medium	Tomato	20	2.0
2 rings	Green pepper	5	0.2
1 tbsp.	Onion, chopped	0	0.1
6 slices	Cucumber	5	0.1
1 tbsp.	French style dressing, low-calorie	15	0
1 slice	Whole wheat bread	50	2.1
12	Grapes	20	0.3
1 cup	Coffee, black	5	0
		360	6.2
SNACK			
1 small	Banana	80	3.2
	Day's total	1200	22.6

DAY 3

BREAKFAST			
1 wedge	Honeydew melon	30	1.3

¾ cup (1.3 oz)	Kellogg's® Raisin Bran cereal	110	4.0
1 slice	Whole wheat toast	50	2.1
1 pat	Butter (or margarine)	35	0
1 cup	Skim milk	85	0
1 cup	Coffee, black	5	0
		315	7.4
LUNCH			
½ cup	Tuna salad	270	0.5
6 leaves	Lettuce	5	0.7
1 small	Apple, with peel	50	2.1
1 cup	Skim milk	85	0
		410	3.3
DINNER			
3 ounces	Turkey, white meat, roasted	150	0
½ cup	Broccoli, chopped	15	3.2
½ cup	Cauliflower	5	1.1
½ cup	Rice, white enriched, long grain	125	0.8
1	Bran muffin	180	3.2
1 cup	Coffee, black	5	0
		480	8.3
SNACK			
½ cup	Strawberries	20	1.7
	Day's total	1225	20.7

DAY 4

BREAKFAST			
½ cup	Orange juice	55	0
⅓ cup (1 oz.)	Kellogg's® All-Bran cereal	70	9.0
1 slice	Whole wheat toast	50	2.1
1 pat	Butter (or margarine)	35	0
1 cup	Skim milk	85	0
1 cup	Coffee, black	5	0
		300	11.1
LUNCH			
	Roast beef sandwich:		
3 ounces	Roast beef, lean	175	0
2 slices	Whole wheat bread	100	4.2
6 strips	Carrots, raw	5	0.8
1 stalk	Celery, raw	5	0.7
1 medium	Pickle, dill	5	1.1
1 medium	Peach	35	1.4
½ cup	Gelatin	70	0
		395	8.2
DINNER			
3 ounces	Chicken, ½ breast, roasted	145	0
½ cup	Green beans	5	2.0
½ slice	Bran banana bread	115	1.8
1 pat	Butter (or margarine)	35	0

½ cup	Pineapple, fresh	35	0.9
1 cup	Coffee, black	5	0
		340	4.7
SNACK			
½ cup	Ice cream, vanilla	135	0
	Day's total	1170	24.0

DAY 5

BREAKFAST			
½ cup	Tomato juice	25	0
⅔	Kellogg's® 40% Bran Flakes cereal	90	3.0
½	Bran banana bread	115	1.8
1 pat	Butter (or margarine)	35	0
1 cup	Skim milk	85	0
1 cup	Coffee, black	5	0
		355	5.8
LUNCH			
	Salad:		
1/6 head	Lettuce	10	1.4
1	Tomato	20	2.0
1 ounce	Ham, lean only	65	0
1 ounce	Cheddar cheese	115	0
½ large	Egg, hard boiled	40	0
½ cup	Bean sprouts	5	1.6
1 tbsp.	Italian style dressing, low calorie	10	0
1 slice	Whole wheat bread	50	2.1
1 pat	Butter (or margarine)	35	0
10 large	Cherries	30	1.2
		380	8.3
DINNER			
½ cup	Minestrone soup	55	1.2
3 ounces	Roast beef, lean	175	0
½ cup	Beets	35	2.1
⅓ cup	Corn	40	3.1
1 medium	Tangerine	30	1.6
1 cup	Skim milk	85	0
1 cup	Coffee, black	5	0
		425	8.0
SNACK			
¼	Cantaloupe	40	1.6
	Day's total	1200	23.7

DAY 6

BREAKFAST			
½	Grapefruit	20	0.6
1 large	Egg, soft, hard, poached	80	0
1	Bran muffin	180	3.2
1 pat	Butter (or margarine)	35	0

1 cup	Skim milk	85	0
1 cup	Coffee, black	5	0
		405	3.8
LUNCH			
½ cup	Tomato juice	25	0
2 ounces	American cheese	210	0
2 slices	Whole wheat bread	100	4.2
1 pat	Butter (or margarine)	35	0
½ cup	Cole slaw	60	1.7
1 cup	Coffee, black	5	0
		435	5.9
DINNER			
3 ounces	Lamb chop, lean, broiled	160	0
½ cup	Spinach	25	5.7
½ cup	Mushrooms	5	0.9
½ cup	Carrots	15	2.3
2 medium	Apricots	20	1.6
1 cup	Skim milk	85	0
		310	10.5
SNACK			
12	Grapes	20	0.3
	Daily total	1170	20.5

DAY 7

BREAKFAST			
½ cup	Orange juice	55	0
⅓ cup	Kellogg's®		
(1 oz.)	Bran Buds® cereal	70	8.0
½ slice	Bran banana bread	115	1.8
1 pat	Butter (or margarine)	35	0
1 cup	Skim milk	85	0
1 cup	Coffee, black	5	0
		365	9.8
LUNCH			
	Turkey sandwich:		
3 ounces	Turkey, white meat	150	0
1 medium	Tomato	20	2.0
2 leaves	Lettuce	0	0.2
1 tsp.	Mayonnaise	35	0
2 slices	Whole wheat bread	100	4.2
½ cup	Strawberries	20	1.7
1 cup	Skim milk	85	0
		410	8.1
DINNER			
½ cup	Apple juice	60	0
3 ounces	Steak, beef	175	0
½ cup	Green peas	40	4.2

½ cup	Rice, white enriched, long grain	125 c.	0.8
1 tbsp.	Onions, chopped	0 c.	0.1
1 cup	Coffee, black	5 c.	0
		405 c.	5.1
SNACK			
1 medium	Peach	35 c.	1.4
	Daily Total	1215 c.	24.4

LEXINGTON 800-Calorie High-Fiber Diet

BREAKFAST
Bran buds 30 g
Skim milk 112 g
Whole wheat bread 25 g
Margarine 8.5 g
1 Multivitiman

NOON MEAL
Navy beans (cooked) 200 g
with ham 5 g
Onion (raw) 12 g
Corn (cooked) 100 g
Brussels sprouts (cooked) 104 g

EVENING MEAL
Tossed salad
Lettuce 50 g
Onion 10 g
Tomato 50 g
Egg (hard boiled) 8 g
Whole wheat muffin 50 g
Margarine 10 g

EVENING SNACK
Graham crackers 15 g

LEXINGTON 1200-Calorie High-Fiber Diet

BREAKFAST
All bran 30 g
Banana 50 g
Skim milk 120 g
Whole wheat bread 50 g,
Margarine 10 g
1 Multivitiman

NOON MEAL
Kidney beans (cooked) 200 g
Brown rice (cooked) 100 g
Carrots 30 g
Celery 30 g
Green beans (cooked) 100 g
Cauliflower (cooked) 100g
Whole wheat bread 25 g
Margarine 9 g

EVENING MEAL
Roast beef 37 g
Potatoes 100 g
Broccoli (cooked) 100 g
Tomatoes, sliced 50 g
Beets (cooked) 100 g

EVENING SNACK
Whole wheat muffin 50 g
Margarine 9 g

August — Week 2

Salad is the dieter's summer staple. It's a good way to get lots of fiber and a minimum of calories. But watch out. Unless you are careful, that salad for lunch can put on more pounds than a sandwich or a blue-plate special.

Slicing meats and cheeses in julienne strips does *not* strip them of their calories. And dressings are loaded with fat. Together, they can add up to "salad slide-back."

A julienne salad—lettuce, radishes, onions, cheese, ham, turkey, dressing, and so on—can run to 775 calories. Not exactly low-cal.

The biggest caloric wallop comes in salad dressings, especially the mayonnaise kind, which can have up to 100 calories per tablespoon. There's lots about this in *All about Mayonnaise,* a free booklet put out by a leading producer, Hellmann's, of Englewood Cliffs, NJ 07632.

The yellowish sauce, originally called bayonnaise or mahonnaise, depending on what legend you hear, is an eighteenth-century French invention. You can understand why a tablespoon "costs" 100 calories when you see the ingredients: "an emulsion of vegetable oil, eggs and/or egg yolks, vinegar, lemon juice, and seasonings." Among the seasonings are salt, sugar, mustard, paprika, and spice oils. Unlike salad dressings, mayonnaise contains no water or flour filler. It is almost pure fat. In this it differs appreciably from salad dressings or imitation mayonnaise, including Miracle Whip, which also contain water and flour filler.

Mayonnaise is rather low in cholesterol and saturated fat, which are associated with eggs, its characteristic ingredient. A tablespoon of mayonnaise contains 10 milligrams of cholesterol, while a large egg contains 252 milligrams, all in the yolk.

Peanut butter has about the same caloric cost—95 calories per tablespoon. You could try sprinkling it on salad greens, as well as putting it in a sandwich. Peanut butter is high in oil, mostly unsaturated. You also get 4 grams of fairly high quality protein per tablespoon, as well as a bit of niacin, phosphorous, and iron, and a respectable amount of potassium. There is even some fiber.

Avocado, a summer salad staple, also is high in fat, the major source of its calories—390 per fruit. But it also gives you as much protein as a breakfast cereal (4 grams) and lots of potassium (2,700 milligrams). Being a natural plant product, it has no cholesterol and only a little saturated fat.

A typical fruit plate is a mound of cottage cheese surrounded by an assortment of juicy hunks of fresh fruit, over which are sprinkled cherries, grapes, or blueberries. Side dishes offer sour cream, a slice of bread, and a pat of butter or margarine. A glass of cool, dry white wine may be at hand. This sort of salad can contain as much as 650 calories.

There are some promising low-cal salads and dressings in the book, *Miracle Cuisine Minceur*, by Ruth K. Malinowski (A&W Visual Library). Here's her Zero-Calorie Salad Dressing, which actually contains a few calories:

½ cup wine vinegar
½ clove garlic, crushed
¼ teaspoon tarragon
1 tablespoon chopped parsley
¼ teaspoon oregano
¼ teaspoon salt

Shake well and pour over salad. This may be stored in the refrigerator for several weeks. Yield: ½ cup.

Here is a handy calories list of common salad ingredients and dressings.

Vegetables	Calories
Artichoke, cooked, base and soft ends	44
Bean sprouts, soya, raw, 1 cup	46
Broccoli, flower stalks, raw, 1 stalk (5½ in. long)	32
Carrots, raw, 1 large or 2 small	42
Cauliflower, raw, 1 cup, flower pieces	27
Celery, bleached, raw, 3 inner stalks or 1 outer stalk	8
Chick peas or garbanzos, ½ cup dried peas	360
Chives, raw, 1 tbsp.	3
Cress, garden, raw, 5 to 8 sprigs	3
Cucumber, raw and not pared, ½ medium	8
Dandelion greens, raw, 1½ cup after cooking	45
Endive, raw, 20 long leaves or 40 small	20
Lettuce, crisphead, iceberg, 3½ oz.	14
Mushrooms, fresh, raw (Agaricus),10 small or 4 large	28
Olives, ripe, canned, 2 large	37
Olives, green, pickled, 2 medium	15
Peppers, green, raw, 1 large empty shell	22
Pickles, cucumber, dill, 1 large	11
Radishes, red, raw, 10 small (1-in. diameter)	17
Spinach, raw, 3½ oz.	26
Tomatoes, ripe, raw, 1 small	22
Turnip, white root, raw, ¾ cup diced	30
Water chestnuts, Chinese, 4 chestnuts	20
Watercress, raw, 10 sprigs	2

Fruit	Calories
Apples, raw, 1 small (2-in. diameter)	58
Avocado, raw, peeled and pitted, ½ (3¼-in. x 4-in.)	167
Blackberries, raw, 1 cup	84
Blueberries, raw, 1 cup	87
Cantaloupe, raw, ¼ melon (5-in. diameter)	30
Cherries, sweet, raw, 15 large or 25 small	70
Fruit cocktail, water pack, ½ cup scant	37
Grapes, American, 22 medium	69
Honeydew melon, raw, ¼ small (5-in. diameter)	33
Loganberries, raw, ⅔ cup	62
Orange, 1 small (2½-in. diameter)	49
Peach, raw, 1 medium	38
Pear, raw, ½ (3-in. by 2½-in.)	61
Pineapple, raw, diced, ¾ cup	52
Plum, damson, raw, 2 medium	66
Raisins, dried, seedless, 1 tablespoon	29
Raspberries, black, raw, ⅔ cup	73
Raspberries, red, raw, ¾ cup	57
Strawberries, raw, 10 large	37
Watermelon, ripe, balls or cubes, ½ cup	26

Dairy Products	Calories
Cottage cheese, creamed, 1 oz., (1 round tablespoon)	30
Process cheese, American, 1 oz.	107
Swiss cheese (Switzerland), 1 oz.	104
Yogurt, made from skim milk 1 cup	122

Fish	Calories
Anchovy, canned, 3 thin fillets	21
Crab with celery salad 3 heaping tablespoons, 2 leaves lettuce	137
Herring, pickled (Bismarck), 3½ oz.	223
Lobster, boiled or broiled, 1 (¾ lb.), 2 tablespoons butter	308
Lobster, canned, ½ cup meat	75
Lobster salad, ½ cup plus 2 leaves lettuce	110
Salmon, canned, 2/5 cup	171
Sardines, Atlantic, canned in oil, 8 medium	311
Shrimp, raw, 3½ ounces	91
Tuna, canned in oil, solids and liquid, ½ cup	288
Tuna, canned in water, solids and liquid, ½ c.	127
Tuna salad, 1 serving	170

Poultry and Meat	Calories
Chicken, canned, boned, 2 tablespoons	151
Hen, stewed, 1 medium thigh, ½ breast	207
Chicken with celery salad, 3 heaping tablespoons, 2 leaves lettuce	185
Turkey, roasted, 1 slice (3 in. by 3 in. by ¼ in.)	80
Bologna, 1 slice (4¼ in. by ⅛ in.)	66
Luncheon meat, 1 slice	81

Salad Dressings	Calories
Blue cheese, 1 tbls.	71
French dressing, 1 tbls.	57
Italian dressing, 1 tbls.	77
Mayonnaise, 1 tbls.	101
Mayonnaise type, 1 tbls.	61
Thousand Island, 1 tbls.	70
Sunflower seeds, ¼ cup	202.5

August — Week 3

Now is the time for all good men (and women) to come to the aid of their muscles.

More accurately, the end of summer is the time to start planning your winter exercise program. If you put it off until fall, then stall some more, you may find yourself snowbound without so much as a jump rope. There are three steps you can take to get yourself in shape *now*.

First, follow the *Dieter's Almanac* Exercise Plan. If you have been on the plan for several weeks, you are already in good shape. If not, start now and by year's end you'll be in top shape. If you're not sure about your condition, see your doctor and take a stress test.

Second, get a book or two on exercise to hype yourself up and get in the mood. (There are some suggestions a few paragraphs farther on.)

Third, join the local YMCA, the Jewish Community Center, or another public exercising facility, or join a private health club.

But before joining a private club, obtain a free copy of *Health Spas: Exercise Your Rights*, from the Bureau of Consumer Protection, Federal Trade Commission, 600 E Street N.W., Washington, DC 20580. There are many legitimate, well-worth-it health clubs and spas around, but there are also some underhanded, outrageously priced ones that put on the pressure and almost force you to sign long-term, expensive contracts.

The FTC receives so many complaints about such spas that it has drafted regulations to control such tactics. For the same reason, some states require spa owners to post bond and put money into escrow to repay customers who are unsatisfied or who are left in their shorts when the spas go out of business.

The federal regulations provide for a cooling-off-period of three days, during which time the new spa member can ask for, and get back, his or her membership money.

The problem is that the spas lure you to a free visit and body analysis, then spend about an hour pitching you for membership for a year, or two years, or three, or for life. The contract is shoved at you, and you are urged to sign. You don't get to take the contract home or to your lawyer to study.

Sign now to take advantage of the "discount"; if you tarry, you pay "full price." Many who sign don't realize they are actually signing papers for a loan, by which they pay out the total membership fee plus a hefty interest.

Before you sign on the dotted line, get answers to these questions:

1. Was everything promised and everything stated by the salesperson put in writing?
2. How long do you have to consider the terms of the contract before signing?
3. Is there a trial period so that you can be sure before you sign?
4. How are the fees paid? Monthly? To whom are they paid—to the club or spa, or to a loan company?
5. What's the place like during busy times—clean, well-maintained, overcrowded? Equipment in good condition? Adequate locker-room facilities and showers?
6. How good are the supervisory and teaching staffs? May you take a class and a workout before joining?
7. How many members? Are there equal facilities for men and women? Any men-only and women-only times on the schedule?
8. Can you get a prorated refund if you become ill or injured or move away or otherwise are unable to use the facilities before your membership expires?

9. Is the facility convenient to home or work? If it's part of a chain, are there reciprocal privileges at other locations?
10. Does it offer child care?
11. What is its experience? That is, how long has it been in the community? What is its track record? Who recommends it? What is the background of the people running it?
12. Can you afford the membership fee? Are there any add-on or special fees for any activities or equipment use?

Here are some good exercise books:

Adult Physical Fitness. Washington, D.C.: U.S. Government Printing Office, 1973.

This slim, useful book is available from the U.S. Government Printing Office, Washington, DC 20402, or from government book stores in Birmingham, Alabama; Los Angeles and San Francisco, California; Denver and Pueblo, Colorado; Washington, D.C.; Jacksonville, Florida; Atlanta, Georgia; Chicago, Illinois; Laurel, Maryland; Boston, Massachusetts; Detroit, Michigan; Kansas City, Missouri; New York City; Cleveland and Columbus, Ohio; Philadelphia and Pittsburgh, Pennsylvania; Dallas and Houston, Texas; Seattle, Washington; and Milwaukee, Wisconsin.

The Fitness Fact Book by Theodore Berland. New York: New American Library, 1981. (Also available from World Almanac, 200 Park Avenue, New York, NY 10017, for $2.50.)

Critical looks at, and evaluations of, sports and exercises.

Aerobics by Kenneth H. Cooper, M.D. New York: Bantam Books, 1968.

The classic on the subject.

Jogging, Aerobics and Diet by Roy Ald. New York: New American Library, 1968.

A sensible program for getting into shape.

The Exerciser's Handbook by Dr. Charles Kuntzleman. New York: David McKay, 1978.

A useful primer on exercising.

The Runner's Handbook by Bob Glover and Jack Shepherd. New York: Penguin Books, 1978.

Read this before you start jogging.

August — Week 4

As you stock wood for the fireplace and oil for the furnace, as you get out the woolens and furs for the cold wind, consider getting an exercise device for those snowbound, homebound, dark days of winter that are sure to come.

Happily, because of the fitness craze, there is a great assortment of home exercising machines to select from. Find a sports store and try out some; work up a sweat on the machines in the display room. Also look at mail-order ads, at the Sears and Ward catalogs, and consult with friends.

A rowing machine simulates the action of rowing a boat. Basically it is a frame that holds two "oars" that pivot and a seat that glides back and forth as you push and pull. If the pull on the oars is adjustable, you can do some real work. Rowing machines exercise only the upper part of the body—essentially arms, shoulders, and chest. Since upper-body exercises raise blood pressure more than lower-body exercises do, rowing machines are not for hypertensive patients.

An exercise cycle, or stationary bicycle, provides a means of exercising the lower part of the body, specifically the thighs. The basic bike is a stand with a front wheel driven with the usual pedals. It has a speedometer to measure speed and record distance and a control knob to increase resistance. You should also be able to pedal backward so as to balance muscle involvement. Fancier bikes tell you, in addition, how many calories you are burning.

Far cheaper than these are simple metal stands that hold your own bicycle, such as are listed in the Sears catalog. You simply place your bike in the stand, adjust the tension on the roller, and pedal away.

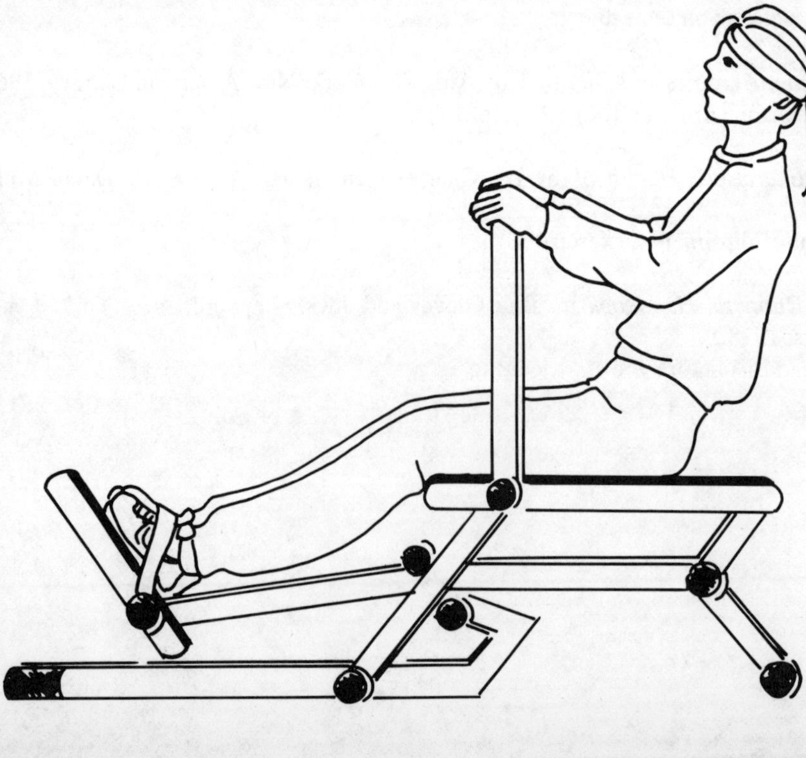

Watch out for home cycles driven by motors. Not only are they more expensive, but they are overrated because it is easy to let the machine do the work instead of your muscles.

Motorized treadmills are worthwhile, however, although they are very expensive: up to $1,000. The principle of a treadmill is that you walk or jog on an endless moving belt. If the belt is driven at a preset speed, you must keep up with it, lose your balance, or get off the machine.

A regular treadmill, powered by foot and kept at an even speed by a heavy flywheel, is just as good. It should have a safety bar at the front for you to hold on to, although some treadmills have wooden rollers under the belt, to allow you to jog without holding on. A built-in feature of some treadmills lets you increase your effort, from running at level to running up a hill. A pedometer tells the distance you have "run." In other models you can increase the workload by adding resistance to the fly-wheel or by raising the incline of the treadmill platform.

There are also jogging pads that provide a soft platform on which your feet can land, which also count your steps, each yard you "travel," in a large readout. Far cheaper is the jogging pad that looks like a black vinyl notepad to which some foam plastic has been cemented. It crudely connects to a mechanical counter. A chart is provided to tell you how many "step strokes" to the mile (880 if your average stride is 36 inches).

Or you can run on a small trampoline.

Cheapest of all is a resilient pad. Jog on it for half an hour every morning.

Finally, there is rope skipping. You can buy all kinds of fancy ropes with counting gadgets attached, but your best bet is a piece of clean clothesline. (Be sure your ceiling is high enough for the rope to clear.)

A last word: Boredom. None of the above will stimulate your mind as it does your body. So put yourself close to a TV or radio set, or wear a stereo headset to help pass the time.

September — Week 1

While Labor Day celebrates the activity of men and women at their jobs, it also could be construed to celebrate the labor of childbirth. Pun aside, this is a good time to examine the nutritional needs of pregnant women.

First and foremost: Pregnancy is *not* the time to diet. While you don't have to eat like a pig if you are pregnant, you should follow the old adage that you are eating for two. Heed the advice of the Committee on Nutrition of the American College of Obstetricians and Gynecologists: "Weight gain during pregnancy should not be restricted unduly, nor should weight reduction normally be attempted. The average weight gain in normal pregnancy is 10 to 12 kg (22 to 27 lb)."

Dr. Roy M. Pitkin, a past chairman of that committee who now heads the Department of Obstetrics and Gynecology at the University of Iowa, points out that "the pattern of weight gain is more important than the total. The optimum is a minimal gain of 1 to 2 kg (2 to 4.5 lb.) during the first trimester, then a steady, linear gain averaging 400 grams (14 oz.) a week until term."

The National Research Council (NRC) points out that the weight gain during the second trimester "involves mainly maternal factors (expansion of blood volume, growth of the uterus and breasts, and accumulation of fat), whereas that of the third trimester reflects principally growth of the fetus and placenta."

Until about the 1970s, doctors tried to keep pregnant patients thin for fear of a condition known as eclampsia, which led to convulsions. Then research failed to support weight gain as a cause of eclampsia. Dr. Pitkin said doctors were confused by true weight gain, which is harmless, and the weight gain caused by edema (accumulation of water), which can be dangerous.

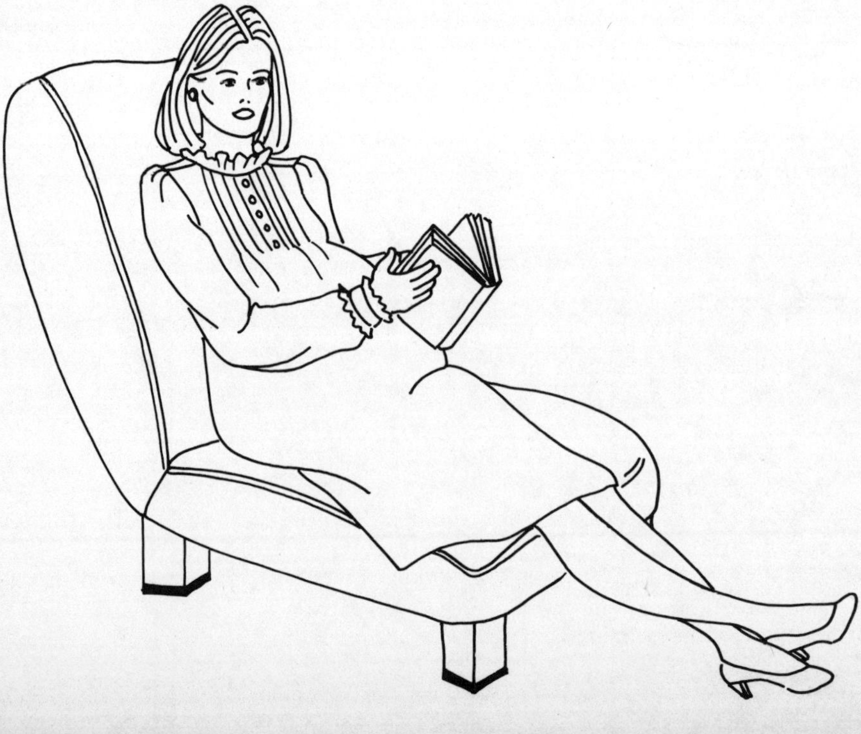

Pregnant mothers shouldn't diet because if they do, they won't get enough essential nutrients, including protein, and because dieting sets up a condition in the body known as ketosis, which can harm the brain of the developing fetus. Women on diets "have children who score less well on IQ tests at age 4," Dr. Pitkin noted.

There is wisdom and good information in the book *What Every Pregnant Woman Should Know* by husband-and-wife team Gail Sforza Brewer and Dr. Tom Brewer (Penguin, 1979). One of the truisms the Brewers drive home is that when mother-to-be diets, so does baby-to-be. And babies who weigh less at birth have a harder start in life than newborn babies of normal weight. The Brewers quote a National Institute of Health study, which points out that "the baby who weighs under 5.5 lb. at birth is more apt to be afflicted with such defects as mental retardation, cerebral palsy, epilepsy, hyperactivity, learning disabilities, respiratory distress syndrome, and sudden infant death syndrome."

Heed these words: "When a mother starts to cut down on her food and salt intake in order not to exceed her doctor's weight limit, she unknowingly begins to starve her unborn baby."

How much food is enough? The Brewers say that a moderately active pregnant woman needs 2,600 calories a day to meet the energy requirements of herself and her baby in the last three months of pregnancy.

To make a baby takes about 80,000 calories, according to NRC estimates. That comes to a daily average of 300 calories that the fetus and the maternal structures need, beyond what the mother needs for her normal activities. The World Health Organization recommends that pregnant women eat 150 calories more every day during the first three months, then 350 calories a day more during the remaining six months. In addition, NRC recommends that pregnant women every day eat 30 more grams of protein and additional amounts of vitamins and minerals (see the Recommended Daily Dietary Allowances table at the back of this book).

Nursing requires lots more nutrition, an additional 750 calories a day. The NRC points out that of 24 pounds gained during pregnancy, 7 pounds is body fat. During three months of breast feeding, this amount of fat can yield 200 to 300 calories a day. That's about a third of the energy cost of breast milk production during this period.

This means that if while nursing you take only an extra 500 calories a day, you will likely be 7 pounds lighter after three months. And if you were overweight at the start of your pregnancy, and want to continue losing weight, you can lose another 7 pounds during the second three months of breast feeding. If you exercise strenuously and regularly, you might be able to lose even more weight.

However, not until you have delivered your baby *and* have stopped nursing should you go on any weight-reducing diet.

September — Week 2

Now that the fun part of summer is over, kids are going back to school. It's a good time to think about the lunches they come home to, take to school, or buy there.

Lunch is perhaps the crucial meal of the day in terms of the child's weight. For most school children, breakfast is a grab and dinner is a bore. But lunch, particularly if eaten in school, is a social activity with classmates.

Dr. Alvin N. Eden points out that walking home for lunch has two advantages: some exercise and a meal you furnish (and control). "Eating lunch in school is another story," he writes in *Growing Up Thin*, written with Joan Rattner Heilman (Berkley, 1975). "If your child brown-bags it, taking lunch with her, don't give her jelly sandwiches and cookies. Prepare a protein sandwich, perhaps tuna fish or chicken, adding a leaf of lettuce or a slice of tomato. Include skimmed milk or fruit juice, a piece of fruit or perhaps some nuts for dessert. Resist tucking in those little surprise packages of potato chips, the can of soda, the lollipops."

Food	Calories
Big Mac	563
Quarter Pounder with cheese	524
Whopper, Burger King	630
Wendy's triple burger	850
Wendy's chili	230
Chicken dinner: 2-piece, Kentucky Fried original recipe	661
Filet-O-Fish, McDonald's	432
French fries	220
Coca-Cola (8 oz.)	96
Chocolate shake	360

Lunch in the school cafeteria can be a problem. What is often offered is high in calories, starches, sugar, and fat, according to Dr. Eden. "Try to influence your youngster to choose as well as possible, and to organize your fellow parents to press for better menu planning."

Your child has even more of a problem if he or she goes down the street with her friends for a fast-food lunch. A burger, fries, and Coke will accumulate as fat on the hips, unless they are accounted for in the child's daily calorie total. The chart at left, from *The Dieter's Complete Guide* (Fawcett Columbine, 1981), gives some examples.

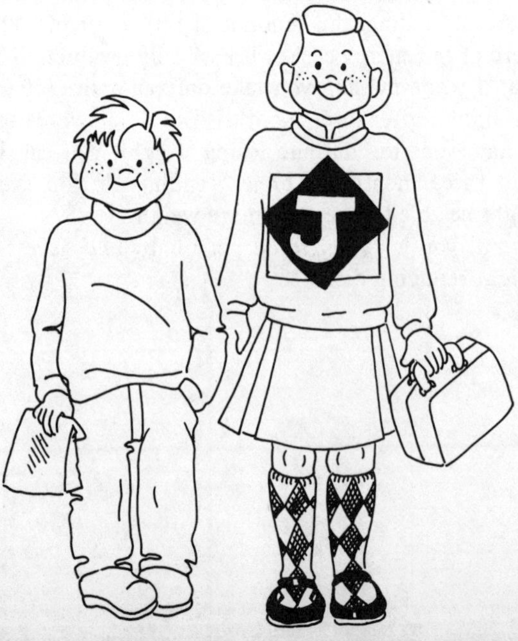

In *The Woman Doctor's Diet for Teen-Age Girls* (Prentice-Hall, 1980), Dr. Barbara Edelstein recommends these lunches.

Sunday: cold chicken, tossed salad with Italian dressing, blueberries, skim milk

Monday: cantaloupe, cottage cheese

Tuesday: open-face tuna salad sandwich, raw vegetables, skim milk

Wednesday: ham-and-cheese sandwich, mustard, pickles, orange

Thursday: open-face turkey sandwich, mustard, lettuce, apple

Friday: yogurt with fresh fruit and raisins

Saturday: chef's salad with strips of cheese and roast beef, Italian dressing, unbuttered corn

If your child tends to be chubby, it's not too early to teach him or her to count calories. Remember, however, that the daily calorie needs of children are far different from yours. And while yours are rather constant, a child's needs change from stage to stage. For example, a 15-pound infant needs 784 calories a day, a 50-pound child needs 1,818 calories, and a 120-pound adolescent girl needs about 2,100 calories to maintain her weight. These data, from the National Research Council, assume a moderate amount of physical activity.

Exercise is especially important in late childhood and adolescence. While babies, toddlers, and small children need proportionally more calories because they are growing at their fastest, teens need to sweat off their baby fat.

Here are the NRC's recommendations for total daily calories for children. If they seem high, it is because they are not diet levels.

	Age	Daily calories
	1-3	1,300
	4-6	1,700
	7-10	2,400
Boys	11-14	2,700
	15-18	2,800
Girls	11-14	2,200
	15-18	2,100

September — Week 3

Millions of the world's people chronically starve for want of enough food. Once a year, about this time, to empathize with their plight and to show some self-sacrifice to God, Jews fast for a day. This is the solemn day of Yom Kippur.

Fasting to reach a holy state is a practice that is thousands of years old. Moses fasted for 40 days and 40 nights before he received the Ten Commandments on Mount Sinai.

Fasting to lose weight is a more recent practice, one that could develop only in our overstuffed modern society. Its intent is to produce, not a state of grace, but a more graceful state, a svelte figure.

There is another important difference. Jews who fast on Yom Kippur, as well as Catholics, yogis, and Buddhists who fast for solemn reasons, generally do so for a day or two and probably do little harm to their bodies. Those who fast to lose weight must do so for months to achieve any results. The health risks are enormous.

A folk tale of fasters says fasting allows the body to rest. Some claim that "fasting brings a welcome physiological rest for the digestive tract and the central nervous system. It normalizes metabolism."

A physician who has done some extensive research in fasting, Dr. Ernst J. Drenick of the Veterans Administration Medical Center in Los Angeles, says that you should not even consider fasting if you are pregnant or breast feeding, or if you have gout, kidney trouble, heart or other circulatory disease, liver disease, anemia, or a nervous disorder.

You have to realize that along with the fat, you are also going to lose a lot of body protein. Much of this will come from shrinking muscles, but you will also lose protein from blood and probably also develop anemia. Your hair will stop growing, and some hair may fall out. Your skin will become dry and scaly.

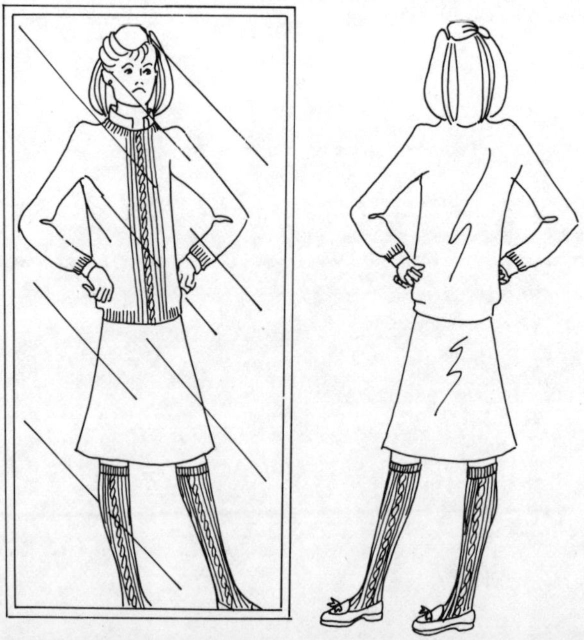

Dr. Drenick's fasters lose about a pound a day, with the fattest patients losing the most, and men losing more than women. The record weight loss was that of a 540-pound man who lost 71 pounds the first month and 40 pounds the second. Very few patients kept their weight off. Of 105 patients, 96 had regained their weight two years later!

Here is some basic information from two standard references: *The Physiological Basis of Medical Practice* by Charles H. Best and Norman B. Taylor (Williams & Wilkins, 1966) and *Principles of Physiology* by David Jensen (Appleton Century Crofts, 1976). Studies of starving people and animals (the difference between fasting and starving is that the first is voluntary) show that profound changes take place in the body within a few days: slowing of metabolism, lowering of body temperature and blood pressure, and slowing of heartbeat.

Initial weight loss is from water loss. Not all the tissues of the body give up their water at the same rates. The first water lost is from reserves. Then healthy tissue starts to break down as water is given up. Muscular tissue, particularly, gives up large proportions of water—about 35 percent of its weight. The heart, being mostly muscle, disintegrates at about the same rate as skeletal muscle.

More than water is lost. During the first phase of fasting, the body easily obtains its energy from carbohydrate in the form of a starch called glycogen, which has been stored in muscles and liver. Since the body carries only a few pounds of glycogen, this energy is soon used up.

Next it turns to its most concentrated form: fat. The body must shift metabolic gears to burn fat for energy instead of the carbohydrate. Because fat burns inefficiently, certain chemical side products, known collectively as ketones, build up. They build up faster in fasting women than in fasting men. No matter the sex, the more a person weighs, the more ketones will accumulate.

Ketones put a load on kidneys and cause acetone breath. The brain and central nervous system, normally powered by sugar, must shift gears too in order to burn ketones for energy. Ketones, a form of alcohol, are probably the reason for "highs" in religious fasts.

At some time before fat stored in the abdomen and under the skin is gone, the body starts stealing protein from muscles (including the heart) and converting it to energy-yielding chemicals. As a result of this loss of protein and fat in supporting tissue, skin hangs and internal organs sag.

Other bad things happen during a prolonged fast:

- Accumulation of fluid in ankles and feet
- Abnormal sensitivity to cold
- Fatigue
- Susceptibility to infection
- Mental changes including apathy, depression, and moral deterioration

Not a pretty picture.

September — Week 4

As fall begins, you begin to pay attention to all those ads telling you and your children to eat breakfast every day, preferably a hot breakfast. And the diet gurus tell you breakfast is the most important meal of the day.

Yet you may hate breakfast. Indeed, it may nauseate you.

Confused? Small wonder. Well, here are the facts.

First, not everyone fasts from dinner to dawn. In fact, most people eat a snack before turning in. If you go to bed late and rise early, there still may be food in your stomach when you awaken.

Second, you have plenty of energy reserves in your body. Glycogen, a starch, is stored in liver and muscles. Your body quickly converts it in order to keep blood-sugar levels up. Then there is fat, oh, so much of it, to be burned or converted to sugar.

Most supporters of hearty breakfasts quote the Iowa Breakfast Study conducted at the University of Iowa in the 1940s and 1950s. It was supported by generous grants from General Mills, a maker of breakfast cereals, and from the Cereal Institute, a promoter of breakfast cereals.

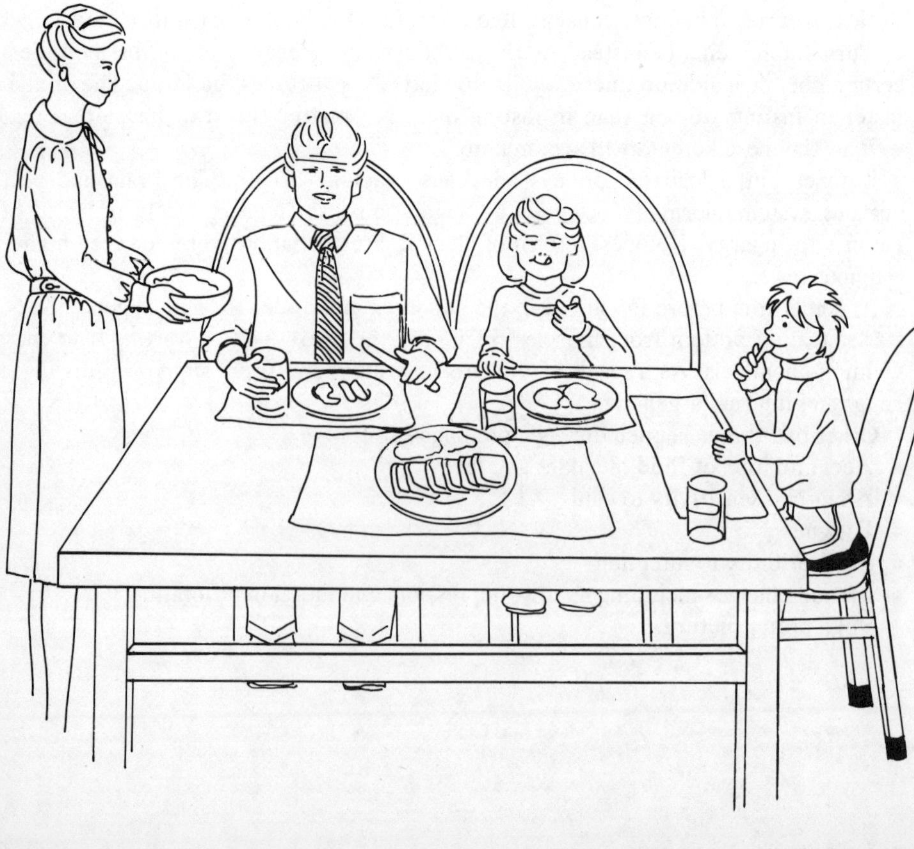

The Iowa research team, led by W. W. Tuttle, reported in 1949 that subjects who ate a light breakfast did better on a stationary bicycle and had quicker reaction times and smaller tremors of the fingers in the morning than when they ate heavy breakfasts or just drank coffee and cream. The light breakfast consisted of fruit, a slice of buttered toast, a glass of milk, and coffee—a total of 400 calories. The heavy breakfast consisted of fruit, cereal and cream, an egg, a slice of bacon, two slices of toast and jam, milk, and coffee—a total of 800 calories.

In studies reported in the 1950s, the Iowans said that when men did not eat anything from 8 P.M. until noon, they had larger tremors and did poorly on the static bicycle, compared to days when they were allowed a basic breakfast of 749 calories (fruit, cereal with sugar and milk, two slices of buttered toast and jelly).

Yet another study, sponsored by the Cereal Institute, found that a cereal-and-milk breakfast produced the same favorable results as a bacon-and-eggs breakfast. (No surprise there.)

However, the researchers found that the omission of breakfast bothered men more often than women. The men said they felt hungry, dizzy, and even nauseated.

And unloved?

The main effect of breakfast seems to be psychological. Unfortunately, the Iowa study did not test for nutrition. It tested style of eating. The researchers should have simply supplied no nutrients, some nutrients, and more nutrients for breakfast if they really wanted to test pure physical reactions.

Listen to Dr. William F. Kremer and Dr. Laura J. Kremer of Maryland. They say that "thin nutritionists who like breakfast" tell us everyone must eat breakfast, that "all that talk about breakfast being necessary to start the day off right is just a lot of hogwash. As a matter of fact, if you are overweight, breakfast is the worst way to start the day."

The Kremers maintain that you are far better off exercising in the morning than eating. It's a better way to boost your metabolism, tone your muscles, sweep the cobwebs from your brain, and whip up your blood circulation. Jog instead of eating granola.

Typical breakfasts are high in carbohydrates and fats. The carbohydrates are rapidly absorbed and boost your blood sugar. But then the blood sugar plummets, and you get hungry again. This occurs about mid-morning, when you want a doughnut. The caffeine in coffee or tea adds to this effect.

As for the benefits of hot cereal versus cold—again, they are psychological. Hot cereal, cold cereal, and bread have an almost identical nutritional content. Actually, the milk added to cereal has more nutrition. Together, cereal and milk about equals bacon and eggs. (If you use skim milk, you save lots of fat and calories.)

This is all by way of emphasizing that a diet has to fit your lifestyle. Unless it does, it is doomed to fail. After a few weeks, you'll be back at your old habits. Better to adjust a diet to you than you to a diet. What counts are the day's total calories. If you prefer not to eat breakfast, don't. If you prefer to eat a light breakfast, do it. Don't let any diet push you around.

October—Week 1

Many people mistakenly believe that World Series fever is produced by the combination of media hype and the fans' excitement over the contest.

Wrong.

World Series fever is the direct result of overeating. You've been stuffing your mouth all season, at games, in front of the TV set, or both. And the more exciting the game, the more calories you packed away, in direct proportion.

Now, with the climax of the season here, you are in crisis, as in any disease. And crisis brings fever. No matter that your team didn't win a pennant. You still favor one of the teams that did, and you want it to beat the other team.

If you're lucky enough, or rich enough, you can actually go to a World Series game. Otherwise, like most fans, you'll watch the games on the tube. Either way, you'll eat enough to be overcome by The Fever. What else could you expect, considering all that you've packed away during the season?

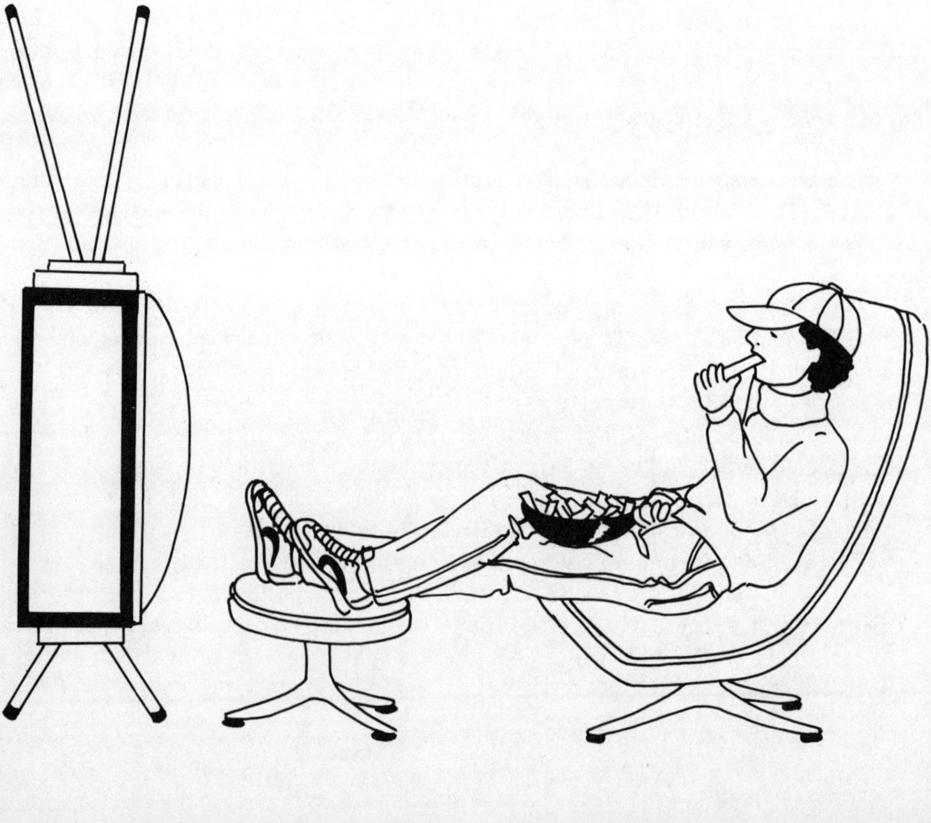

Think of it this way:

1. Ball fields are merely giant open-air restaurants designed so that eaters can watch a ball game.
2. Ball games on TV aren't free; you're paying for them by guzzling the beer and eating the foods hawked by the advertisers who put the games on the air.

Look at the game situation first.

Even before the team warms up, lines form in front of the food stands, the beer stands, the peanut stands. And hawkers shout their wares from the aisles.

There is that technique, seen only at sporting events, in which food is passed from hand to hand in one direction down a row of baseball fans. Then money travels back the other way. Often, too, change comes back, hand to hand.

The litter that remains after a ball game is testimony to the eating compulsion. Few can resist the smell of peanuts or popcorn or red hots as the sphere flies through the air.

In case you want to watch calories as closely as you watch the pitcher, here are some data.

Food	Calories	Protein	Fat	Carbohydrates	Cholesterol
Hot dog	170	7.5 g	13.5 g	1.3 g	34 mg
Bun	119	3.3	2.2	21.2	7
Relish	20	—	—	5.0	—
Mustard	4	0.2	0.2	0.3	—
Peanuts (10)	105	4.7	8.8	3.7	—
Potato Chips (10)	115	1.0	8.0	10.0	—
Popcorn	82	1.8	4.0	10.6	70
Beer	150	1.0	—	14.0	—
Coke	145	—	—	—	—
Coffee	35	—	1.0	6.5	—
Creamer	20	—	2.0	2.0	—
Totals	965	19.5	37.7	74.7	111.0

Now for the game on TV. It is even more dangerous because all that beer and food is there, within reach, or but a few steps away. So here are a few rules to help you concentrate on the game and not on the goodies.

1. Never sit down to a game on an empty stomach. Always make sure you have eaten a meal before starting to consume a game. With your stomach satisfied, your nervous snacking will be delayed at least for a couple of innings.

2. Do *not* watch the game in the kitchen. There's enough food there to kill you.

3. Don't put peanuts, candy, or other high-calorie goodies in the den or whatever room you're in. Make it an effort to get up and fetch such foods.

4. Do stock the TV room with lots of slices of apples, pears, carrots, celery, a huge bowl of unbuttered, unsalted popcorn made without oil in a hot-air popper, plenty of diet soda, and a full pot of coffee or tea.

5. During the seventh-inning stretch, and when you have to use the toilet, don't walk through the kitchen.

Good luck. These suggestions won't relieve the fever, but they should prevent that sick feeling you would otherwise get when you step on the scale after the championship game.

October—Week 2

In honor of Columbus Day, embark on a voyage of self-discovery. Take this quiz and see how smart a dieter you are. Below are 10 statements. Each is followed by a *T* or *F*. Circle *T* if you believe the statement is true, *F* if you believe it is false.

Ready? Go!

1. The best way to lose weight is to eat lots of protein and little or no carbohydrate. **T F**
2. Playing tennis will make me thin. **T F**
3. Fruits like pineapple and grapefruit contain special enzymes that melt fat. **T F**
4. Diets are too complicated; I'll succeed if I just cut back. **T F**
5. I can fill up with all the coffee I want. **T F**
6. Slow metabolism makes most people fat. I probably have a bad thyroid. **T F**
7. I'll save lots of calories on my diet by giving up red meat. **T F**
8. Fasting is absolutely the best way to lose weight. **T F**
9. Pizza is one of the worst junk foods there is. **T F**
10. Margarine has fewer calories than butter. **T F**

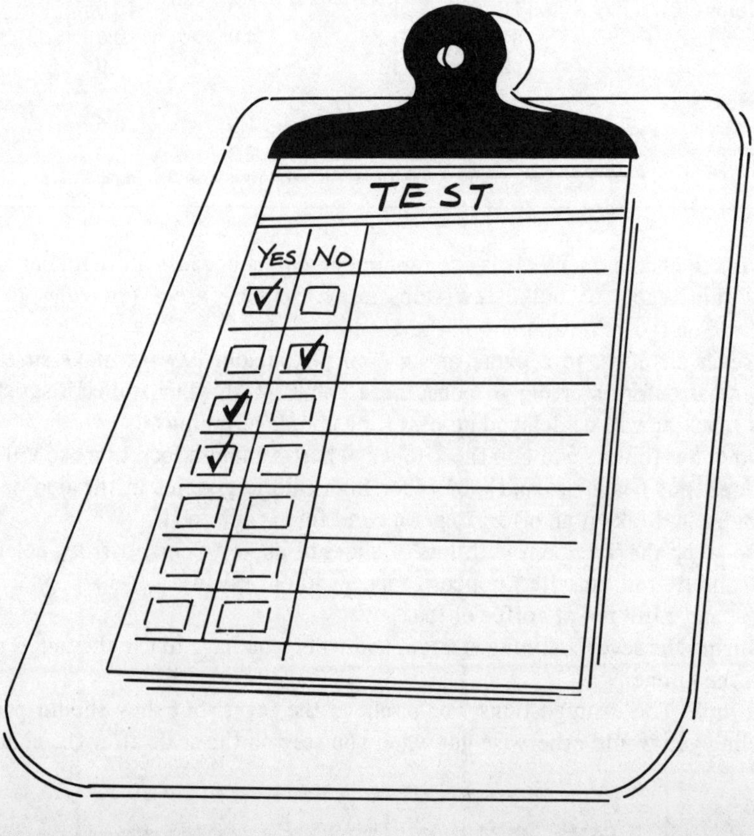

Answers: All 10 statements are False. If you scored 10 correct, you are a Perfect Dieter. A score of 8-9 makes you a Nearly Perfect Dieter, 6-7 is Average, 4-5 is a Deluded Dieter, 2 - 3 is Foolish Dieter, and 0-1 is a Dummy Dieter. Explanations follow.

1. Despite protein's white-hat status, it is not any less fattening than carbohydrate. Both "cost" about 4 calories per gram. Your body needs about the same quantity of each: around 60 grams a day. The real villain is fats, which cost 9 calories per gram.

2. Tennis is a good game and a mildly active sport, but you'd have to play 8.3 hours to lose a pound. This is because you have to burn 3,500 calories less than you eat to lose a pound of body fat. Tennis burns 420 calories per hour.

3. This phony statement is the basis of the Beverly Hills Diet and those sleazy pass-around-the-office diets sometimes labeled the Mayo Diet or the Rockefeller Diet. Fruit is a good low-calorie snack, but it contains no magical enzyme.

4. Just cutting back is meaningless. Back from what? To what? Like any difficult endeavor, you need a plan and you need to stick to it. Otherwise you merely fool yourself.

5. Coffee is not without calories. According to Dr. Samuel Natelson, former chairman of the Biochemistry Department at Michael Reese Hospital, a cup of black coffee contains 50 calories. "Think of it as coffee bean soup," he says.

6. Very few people have faulty metabolism—perhaps fewer than 10 percent. There is probably nothing wrong with your thyroid gland. Still, there are diet doctors who put their overweight patients on thyroid hormone to speed up their metabolism and thus burn off a little more fat. But the hormone has its dangers, especially for persons with susceptible heart conditions—known or unknown. You can greatly increase your metabolic rate, and hence the burn-off of fat, simply by exercising. When you've worked up a sweat, you'll know you've upped your metabolism. It's the safest way.

7. You can live very nicely without red meat, mainly beef. While it is an excellent source of protein, beef is riddled with fat. But that doesn't mean you'll lose weight. If you replace the beef with leaner meats (that is, muscle food) such as poultry and fish, you'll still be getting plenty of fats along with your protein. And mode of preparation has a lot to do with it. Frying adds many calories because of the oil. Broiling and barbecuing are best because they allow much of the fat to drip off.

8. For the first week or so, you'll lose lots of weight by fasting. But any fast that lasts longer than a day or two is dangerous. Your body will be in a severe state of stress, much like the railroad engineer trying to keep a steam engine going after the fuel has run out. He starts hacking up the extra cars behind for wood for the fire. Similarly, your body in starvation steals fuel from likely internal sources: first the fat, then muscle protein, including the muscle of the heart.

9. Pizza has been bad-rapped for too long. It is an excellent food, containing as it does nutrients from four food groups: cereal, in the crust; dairy, in the cheese; vegetable, in the tomato sauce and mushrooms; and meat, in the sausage. Pizza's problem is that it tastes so good you can't stop at one slice!

10. Margarine and butter are both fats, and both give 7.2 calories per gram, or about 100 calories per tablespoon. Made from vegetable oils, margarine has an advantage in that it contains no cholesterol and less saturated fats than butter, which is made from milk. Diet or imitation margarine has fewer calories because it contains water, which dilutes the fat and consequently the calories per tablespoon.

October—Week 3

In the dark days before electricity and refrigeration and jet airplanes, long-distance travelers had to be very cunning if they were not to starve to death en route. They packed food that was dried and salted. For them, the taste of the food was much less important than the necessity of the food for survival. Travel over the oceans was even more hazardous than overland travel. Columbus, the Pilgrims, and others who ventured over from Europe were hardy indeed to survive in those wood-planked square-riggers.

Even hardier were the Polynesian explorers who undertook expeditions in the Pacific Ocean. They left their island homes in relatively small craft that were open to the elements and had little room to store coconuts, papaya, and other food. Neither was there any certainty they would find food on the land they set out for so many weeks or months ago.

Since they could not pack their nutrition in their dugouts or on their rafts, they packed it on their bodies in the form of fat. That's the conclusion of Dr. George F. Cahill, Jr., and a team of anthropologists at Harvard University. They believe that the human ability to overeat—that is, to eat even when not hungry—has enabled our species to survive sieges, migrations, famines, droughts, and even ice ages. But what was good for times of scarcity is bad for times of abundance.

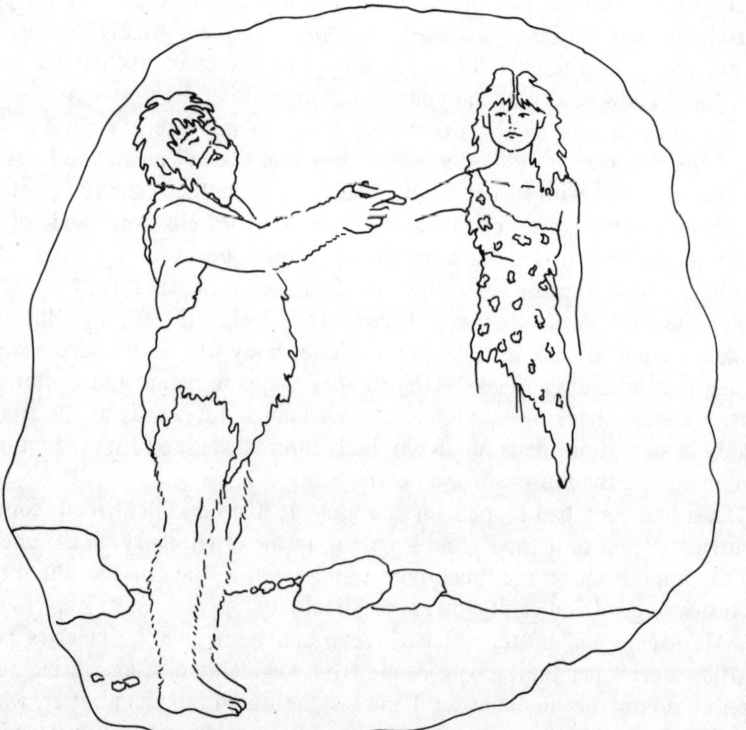

Dr. Cahill, who is a professor of medicine at Harvard and treats contemporary overeaters, observed that ancient people were a lot smarter than we are. They knew how to use food, rather than let food use them.

For example, the Polynesian explorers deliberately gorged themselves until they each weighed about 250 pounds. They overate to accumulate fat on their bodies. The fat enabled them to survive the ordeal of hunger. The fat contained energy and water, the two life-sustaining substances that would not be available in food during the months they would be at sea.

Fat also helped dwellers of ancient walled cities survive in war. They stuffed themselves as armies surrounded them to lay siege. Body fat is a "beautiful tool of survival," in Dr. Cahill's view.

Animals use fat to survive too. The hummingbird eats ravenously so that its weight doubles before it takes off on its annual migratory flight across the Gulf of Mexico. The black bear eats everything in sight in preparation for its long winter's sleep.

There is a difference between animals driven by instinct to overeat at certain times of the year and us. We civilized human beings overeat for other reasons. Our brain overrides any signals from the body that it has had enough to eat, thank you.

You don't eat because you are hungry, or because some instinct drives you to, or because you *need* to. You eat because you *want* to.

This control of eating by brain rather than body is unique to human beings. That is why people get so fat and wild animals do not, and why eating experiments with laboratory animals have little or no relation to human beings.

This is also why there is no use blaming hormones or metabolism for your weight gain. According to Dr. Cahill, you'll lose weight, and you'll keep it off, only when you realize that *you*, not some mysterious forces, control your eating behavior.

You stuff your body with excess food for reasons of emotions or habit. Instead of eating when your body tells you to—as animals do—you eat by the clock, or on command of others (parents, spouse, dinner companion, TV commercial), or when you emotionally feel you need balm and solace (when lonely, bored, frustrated, angry, depressed).

In other words, you eat on signal from external sources in your environment rather than from internal signals in your body. If the food is there, you eat it. Not because you are hungry. Look at the buffet, for instance, and see how you overeat. Like the mountain to the climber: It is there.

For these reasons, Dr. Cahill called obesity "one of the most challenging problems in medicine, similar to that of drug addiction." As for its cure, he is pessimistic of all treatments other than simple, direct intellectual control of eating. In other words: willpower. You have to exercise the same control to stop eating that ancients exercised to gorge in order to survive.

No one ever said it was easy to lose weight. No one ever said that life is fair. The sooner you realize both these truths, the sooner you'll be slim.

October—Week 4

If you love to skate and ski in the winter, you should start preparing yourself *now*.

Dr. Richard H. Dominguez of Central DuPage Hospital, Winfield, Illinois, advises that speed and figure skating are excellent conditioning sports, but tough on ankles. Also, he notes that "cross country skiing is the single best exercise activity available to modern man[and woman]. Obviously the sport has limitations of climate and season, but as an overall fitness activity and a beautiful way to see a winter landscape it is unsurpassed."

In *The Complete Book of Sports Medicine* (Scribner's, 1979) Dr. Dominguez cautions: "Cross country skiing is considered by many to be a perfectly safe sport, but it isn't. Injuries do occur, mostly when going down ice slopes, and they can be serious. This sport is not recommended for people with heart trouble who are not in excellent condition and have not been cleared by a physician. It is not recommended for asthmatics."

Dr. Kenneth G. Campbell of Palo Alto Medical Center, California, observes that skiing has become especially popular among adults 21 to 55 years of age. "Proper training is again an important factor in reducing injuries; less skilled skiers have higher injury rates than do more highly skilled skiers. Because skiing is an endurance sport, adequate conditioning is essential to prevent fatigue-related injuries." He suggests a preseason conditioning program.

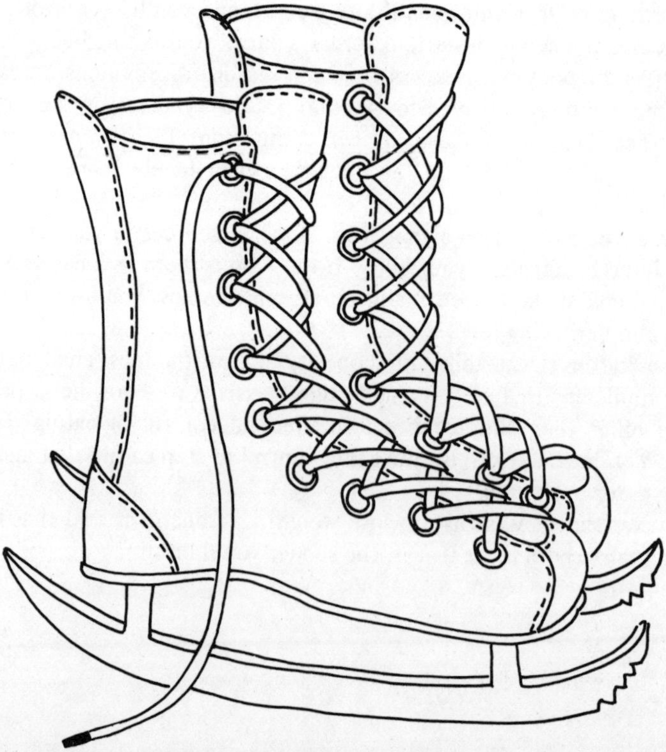

The first phase of your winter sports preseason conditioning program should be to get, and stay, physically fit. (The *Dieter's Almanac* Exercise Plan is a good way to accomplish these goals. If you have been on it, fine. If not, you should start now; by mid-January of next year you'll be in top shape.)

Once you are in shape, get a copy of *Caldwell on Cross Country* (Stephen Greene Press, 1975). It will tell you everything you need to know about training for cross country (called X-C by its fans). The author is John Caldwell, credited with introducing this oldest of snow sports to the North American public.

Some elements of Caldwell's conditioning program include:

1. *Distance training.* This means jogging, hiking, biking, rowing, and roller-skiing. Depending on how serious you are, you should take up one or more of these activities and learn to sustain and pace yourself. Caldwell recommends workouts of from 40 minutes to 3 hours.

2. *Uphill running.* One technique is to walk in strides similar to those used in X-C, with or without poles.

3. *Arm pulls.* Use elastic bands or weights to improve the strength and technique of your poling action.

4. *Strength training.* Sit-ups, back-ups, chin-ups, and weight lifting all strengthen the right muscles; so does running in the surf.

As for downhill skiing, here are some tips from Dr. Laurence E. Morehouse of the Human Performance Laboratory at the University of California, Los Angeles. In *Maximum Performance*, which he wrote with Leonard Gross (Simon and Schuster, 1977), Morehouse writes: "The emphasis on conditioning should be on the lower body, but the upper body shouldn't be neglected." His recommendations: side-to-side jumping, heel and toe raises, step-ups or bench stepping, kangaroo hops, half-squats, push-ups, arm curls, and distance training.

Ice skating requires a fitness program that emphasizes strength and flexibility. Unlike X-C, it is not a sport most people can take up in middle age. That is, you probably shouldn't take it up, you should go back to it. Follow the rule that only adults who ice skated as children should do so in late life, and you'll be safe.

Dr. Morehouse's training suggestions include some of the same exercises you use to prepare for jogging: upside-down bicycle pedaling, sprinter's stretch, heel-cord stretch, toe-touch, and knee hugs. Also, side-to-side jumping, heel and toe raises, steps-ups, kangaroo hops, and half-squats.

He adds that "to skate fast, you must learn to relax your muscles." Yoga and meditation can help. So can sessions of just sitting or lying and concentrating on relaxing each and every muscle.

All four winter sports—figure and speed skating, downhill and X-C skiing are good aerobic exercises. Below are some data. But first, some advice. Don't replenish and overstock the number of calories you burn on the ice or trails. When you get back to the lodge or warmup shack, you will be tempted to down a cup of hot cocoa, hot toddy, or buttered rum. There's lots of calories in them cups! If you want a warming, no-calorie drink, try a cup of hot spiced tea. A cinnamon stick adds class.

Here are those calories, taken from *The Fitness Fact Book* (New American Library, 1980).

Sport	Calories per Minute
Cross-country skiing (7.5 mph)	15.8
Cross-country skiing (5 mph)	12.0
Downhill skiing (10 mph)	10.0
Cross-country skiing (3 mph)	9.0
Ice skating (10 mph)	6.6

October—Week 5

Halloween is a diet disaster. The haunting ghosts of fattening foods fly in and hover just as certainly as the school-age goblins toddle from house to house.

It is no accident that this evil night falls just before the first of November, the start of the long, cold, barren part of the year.

Sophisticated as we think we are, we are still guided by primitive motivations, even as we approach the beginning of the twenty-first century. Those little goblins dressed as witches, "E.T.," and other fantastic beings are our reaffirmation that there is nothing to fear in the dark. Perhaps that's true. But there is much to fear from the treats that are given out. They are carbohydrate and calorie disasters.

Into the children's bags are dropped Mary Janes, Three Musketeers, Snickers, Hershey bars, lollipops, cookies, jawbreakers, sticks of chewing gum, caramel cubes, and popcorn balls. The evil abroad on Halloween is the notion that sweets are treats. It is another of society's sanctions that food is a useful means of dealing with emotions. It is akin to the message we give infants with their bottle: Eat, eat. You'll feel better.

Now at each door is a stockpile of goodies, ready to be plucked and dropped into the goblin's bag. (Of course, if it's a slow night and some of the stock remains, Mommy gets to treat herself!)

On Halloween, the treat is the trick. Rather than pull a prank on any home that refuses to offer sweets, the children are subjected to the Diet Prank. They are tricked into believing that sweets are neat, that fears can be overcome by food, that the risk of being abroad on the night of evil is worth it. And the winner of the night is the boy or girl who has harvested the most and the best treats.

What is a parent to do? While Halloween has status neither as a religious event nor as a national holiday, it persists. It is resuscitated every year by the commercial interests that make, advertise, and sell the sweets and the costumes. There's no use trying to ignore Halloween. Instead, you have to plan for it.

Meet with your neighbors and see if they'll go along with a new kind of Halloween treat. Instead of candy and cookies, why not drop fruit into the trick-or-treat bag? Apples, pears, oranges, bananas. Better yet are nonfood treats. You might consider giving something a child would like. Some suggestions: a patch (sew-on or iron-on), a key chain, a coloring book, a color pencil or pen, next year's calendar, a small toy, a flower.

If you're planning a Halloween party, beware of those evil standbys loaded with calories. Every doughnut costs you 170 calories or more. Apple cider is 120 calories a glass. Pumpkin pie, at a whopping 275 calories per average wedge, at least gives you a respectable amount of Vitamin A for all its evil. And watch out for the three empty P's: pretzels, popcorn, and potato chips. (They are empty because you get nothing from them but calories.)

When you think of witches, think of Giles Cory, the only person in American history ever sentenced to death by pressing. Onto Farmer Cory were piled stones and boulders. Defiant until the end in the madness of Salem, Massachusetts, in 1692, his last words reverberate through the centuries as a curse:

"More weight! More weight!"

November—Week 1

Like the dentist who teaches you to brush and floss your teeth every day, Dr. R. Philip Smith seems to be hurting his future business. He is medical director of La Costa, the world's largest spa, located near San Diego, California, and known as an attraction for the richest and the most famous. The facilities offer a luxurious assortment of physical activities. On the immaculately kept grounds are a professional golf course, several huge outdoor pools, some indoor pools, a jogging track, tennis courts, and gyms. These facilities, plus the low-cal gourmet meals and the service and pampering are what attract those who can afford it.

Still, says Phil Smith, who left his surgical practice and a professorship in Seattle to join La Costa, you don't need all this in order to keep fit. Moreover, he stresses, you neither have to sweat nor compete with anyone else. "Exercise can be pleasant and enjoyable, and it doesn't have to take more than 10 to 14 minutes each day. In fact some exercises can be performed while going about ordinary routine tasks." His *The La Costa Diet and Exercise Book* (Grosset & Dunlap, 1977) offers clever little exercises to do during your other daily activities.

(These exercises don't conflict with the *Dieter's Almanac* Exercise Plan. You can do both. If you haven't started that program, there is no time like now. Begin this week to be in top shape for Valentine's Day.)

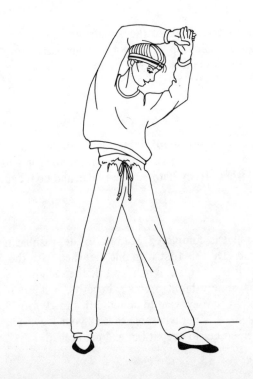

Here is a selection of Dr. Smith's exercises.

Stretch

In the morning when you wake up, before you get out of bed, simply stretch. Stretch to your full ability and yawn as wide as you can. This is what a cat or a dog does after it has been sleeping, and it ought to come naturally to you too. Stretch and enjoy it, with your arms, your legs, your entire body.

Toe Touch

It is now time to get out of bed. After you swing your feet over onto the floor, do not get up immediately. Sit on the edge of the bed and bend over and touch your toes four or five times. Then stand up and stretch as high as you can, as if you were trying to touch the ceiling. Continue to stretch for a count of 10 to 20.

Jog in Place

On your way into the bathroom for your morning toilet, pause to run in place for a count of about 100 steps. As you improve, you can gradually build this to 200. Raise your knees as high as you can without pain. Do not worry if you get slightly out of breath. The object of this exercise is to get your pulse rate up to 120.

Toe-Up

As you brush your teeth and go about the remainder of your toilet, you can exercise your calves and ankles by rising up and down on your toes. You should be able to do anywhere between 45 to 75 toe-ups. As you perform this exercise, try to remember to keep your abdominal muscles tight.

Bumps

As you shave or put on your makeup, tighten your abdominal muscles and roll your pelvis forward, making sure to keep your gluteus maximus (or buttock) muscles tense. Hold for counts of anywhere from 25 to 50; then relax and do it again.

Leg Lift

When your morning toilet is completed, hold on to the washbasin again and do six or eight leg lifts and twists. Do this first with one leg, then with the other, pointing your toes inward for a few lifts, then straight forward, then slightly outward. You do not have to lift the leg extremely high to obtain benefits; just lift it as high as you can comfortably. Eventually you may want to increase this to 10 to 15 lifts with each leg. If you have a back problem, it is not advisable to kick your legs backward. Whether your back is weak or not, remember to keep it flat and not arched.

Body Twist

In the shower, spread your legs apart, securing your feet against the sides, keeping your stomach tight. Bend your elbows, and twist your torso back to the right so that your right elbow reaches behind your back. Then twist to the left. Repeat six or eight times. This benefits the shoulders, waist, and abdomen.

Instead of having coffee in the middle of the morning or in the afternoon, try an exercise break. It is just as refreshing and has more long-range benefits. Here are some suggestions.

Wall Push-Up

Stand about two feet from the wall, place your hands on the wall for support, and then lean. Push yourself back and forth from the wall 10 or 15 times. This will help the muscles of your shoulders and upper arms. As you adjust to this exercise, you can increase the number of times you do it. You can add further benefits by placing your hands so that the fingers of each hand point in toward each other. Or you can stand a little farther back from the wall so that you add more weight onto your arms. A variation of the wall push-up can be done at your desk. Standing a few feet from the desk, rest your hands on the edge and do your push-ups.

Leg Press

An excellent desk exercise is to cross your legs and press them against each other. This can be done in two variations. With your legs crossed at the thighs, and with them crossed at the ankles or calves, the pressure can be directed forward and backward. This exercise is excellent for thighs, buttocks, and abdomen.

Body Lift

Another exercise that can be done seated at your desk involves leaning forward slightly with your feet lightly on the floor and your hands on the arms of the chair, and pushing up. The object is to lift yourself from the chair using your arms and shoulders. In the beginning, you may have to help yourself along by using your feet, but eventually you should be able to lift yourself entirely with your arms, 8, 10, or even 20 times.

Take the Stairs

Do not depend so much on the elevator. If you are 20 or 30 floors up, of course you have to use the elevator—but only part of the way. Get off a few stops below your floor and walk up the rest of the way. In the beginning, you should try only two or three flights, but you can add a flight every few days or every few weeks.

November — Week 2

Although modern science has accomplished some amazing things—such as placing a man on the moon and manipulating chromosomes—appetite and weight control are almost as mysterious today as they were a century ago. The best that can be said is that scientists are studying them at long last.

The findings are like pieces here and there in a jigsaw puzzle. While the picture is far from complete, here are 10 findings. Perhaps some will offer new insights to your own struggle with overweight and overeating.

1. Human beings regulate body weight as precisely as animals do, maintaining it within narrow limits over extended periods. Unlike animals, observed Dr. Richard E. Keesey of the University of Wisconsin, Madison, "the set-points in human beings vary to a much greater degree." Oddly, "obese individuals maintain and defend their body weight in the same fashion, and as effectively, as an individual of normal weight."

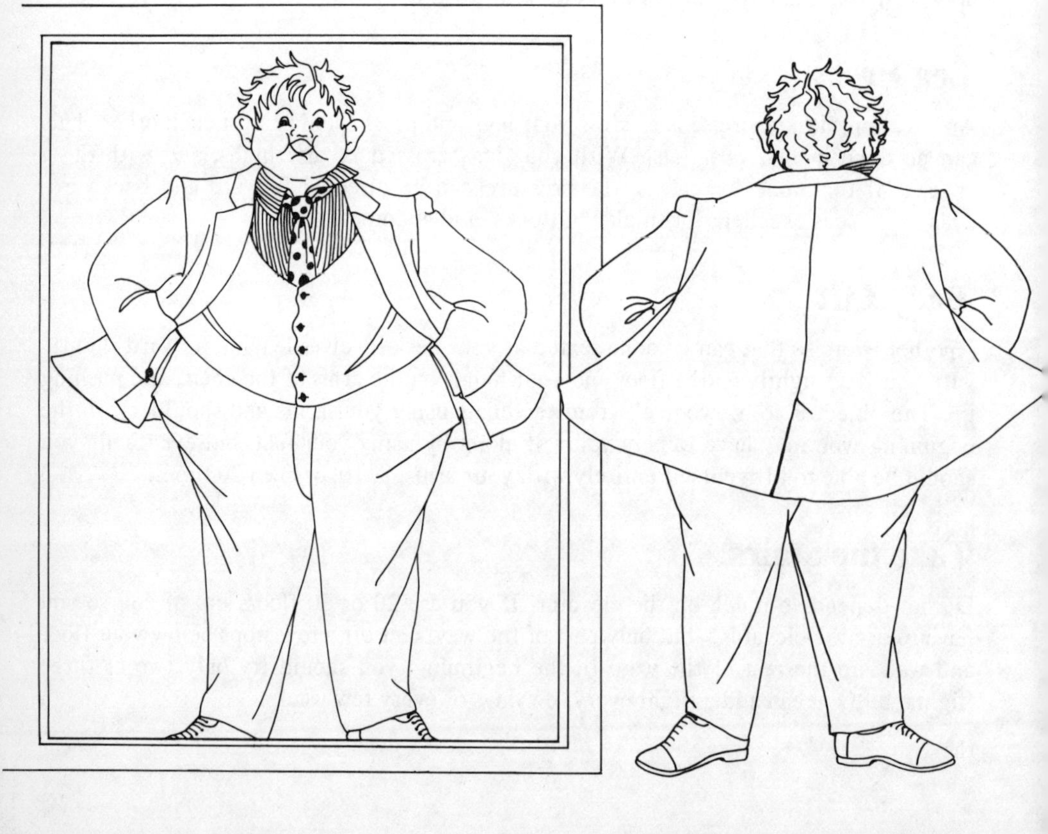

2. Appetite is regulated by a primitive part of the brain known as the hypothalamus. Drs. Luis Hernandez and Bartley G. Hoebel of Princeton University found that when this part of the brain was stimulated by nerve chemicals known as adrenergics, appetite was satisfied. When other chemicals known as dopamines prevailed, appetite was sharpened. They postulated that the amount of fat on the body determines which chemicals are released. But they didn't know why fat content differs so in different people.

3. Zinc has a lot to do with appetite. Dr. Robert I. Henkin of Georgetown University Medical Center, Washington, D.C., found that in laboratory animals and in people, zinc depletion was associated with both loss of appetite and loss of taste. Treatment with zinc sulfate restored both in patients who had diseases that caused the zinc depletion. As for those with too much appetite and too good taste, cutting zinc from the diet is no answer. That mineral is essential to several normal bodily functions. (For more information, see the *Dieter's Almanac* guide to Vitamin and Minerals in this book.)

4. The contours of your body are shaped by deposits of fat. The way it accumulates here and there was determined by your genes before you were born, according to Dr. Ronald K. Kalkhoff, chief of the TOPS Medical Research Program at Milwaukee County Medical Complex. That's why your figure is probably like that of one of your parents or grandparents or an aunt or uncle.

5. However, the total of fat on your body is largely determined by outside factors. It starts before birth. According to Dr. Kalkhoff, if your mother ate heavily while you were still in the womb, especially toward the end of the pregnancy, then overfed you when you were an infant, she helped increase the number of progenitor cells that later would become fat cells on your body.

6. There are sexual differences regarding the locations of the major fat deposits. Overweight women tend to accumulate fat below the waist, specifically on lower abdomen, hips, thighs, and buttocks. Overweight men tend to accumulate fat above the waist, on their chests and stomachs.

7. Dr. Kalkhoff believes that heavy spots can be trimmed down. Dieting helps reduce total fat. Exercise is more selective. It trims fat over muscles, such as at the abdomen and thighs. Exercise can't help trim breasts, which are accumulations of fat tissue around glandular tissue. The usual problem with exercising in middle age is that by the time you decide to do it, decades of inactivity have slipped by, your muscles have gone lax, and you find calisthenics difficult, if not impossible.

8. Knowing you have inherited the tendency to have larger than average breasts, belly, buttocks or thighs doesn't mean you need give up. According to Dr. Kalkhoff, diet and exercise have a three to four times greater influence over your figure than heredity does.

9. Crash diets that produce quick weight loss take more water than fat off your body. Ditto diet pills. As for massage, says Dr. Kalkhoff, "no matter how hard you squeeze or hit a pound of butter you'll still have a pound of butter." To reduce its mass, you have to "burn" it.

10. "More body fat and less lean tissue are lost when diet and exercise are combined than when diet is used alone," wrote Drs. Albert J. Stunkard and Kelly D. Brownell of the University of Pennsylvania in *Obesity* (Saunders, 1980). "Changes in body weight cannot be explained solely by the increase in caloric expenditure due to exercise. Exercise may promote weight loss through a decrease in appetite (and) increase in basal metabolism."

November — Week 3

It's bad enough that we pay tribute to the Pilgrims by gorging ourselves. What's worse is that the modern version of the Thanksgiving feast is devastating to anyone trying to lose weight.

A typical Thanksgiving dinner gives you a total of almost 2,000 calories, which come largely as carbohydrates and fats. You also get a smashing 259 milligrams of cholesterol.

It is easy to achieve this dietary disaster even with moderate portions. Making up the total are one Scotch on the rocks, a wedge of Camembert cheese, some crackers, onion soup, a muffin and butter, 3⅓ ounces of turkey meat (no skin), some stuffing and gravy, candied sweet potatoes, cranberry sauce, salad with French dressing, a glass of dry wine, a slice of pumpkin pie topped by some whipped cream, a handful of walnuts, and coffee with cream and sugar.

Of course, you can save calories by avoiding the drinks, the muffin and butter, the stuffing and gravy, the pie, and the nuts. And by drinking black coffee or unsweetened tea. But it is not likely you will be able to restrain yourself in the company of friends and family who will seem offended by any but a hearty appetite on this festive day.

You *can* celebrate by eating and still watch your diet. Simply follow the plan of the Plymouth Thanksgiving dinner that follows. It is not only better for your diet but also closer to the original celebration.

The first Thanksgiving dinner in 1621 was held, you may recall, at Plymouth Plantation. That is on the bay, and so they served cod, shellfish, and smoked eel as the main courses. You should also serve fish.

The main reason for the holiday was to give thanks to God for their being alive and

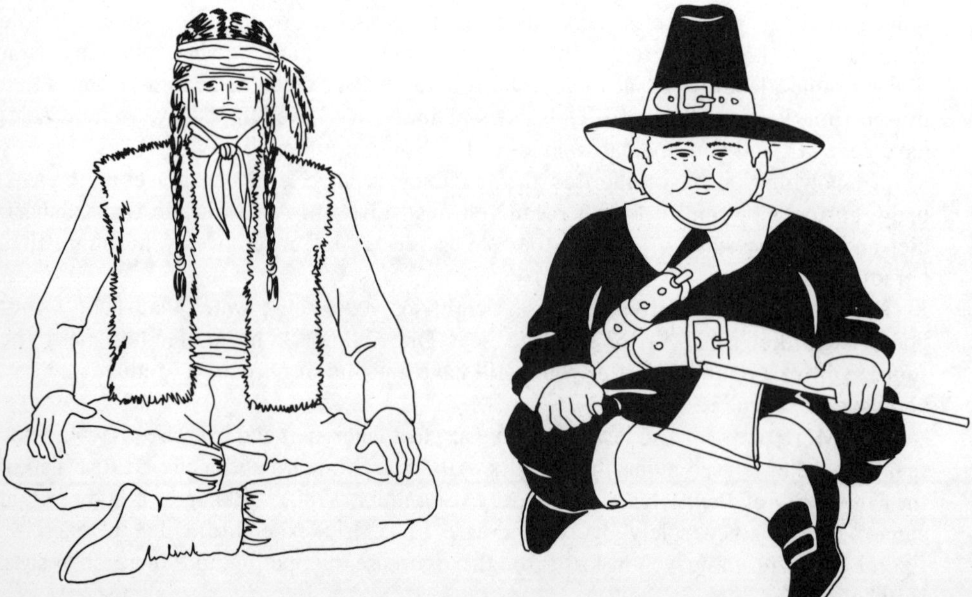

for the bountiful harvest that helped them survive their first winter in the New Land. Since that meant crops such as corn and other vegetables, your Thanksgiving fish dinner should be accompanied by cornmeal bread and succotash (corn and lima beans).

And beer, for not all Pilgrims were teetotalers.

If you don't like beer but still want to have a reconstructed Plymouth dinner, have some sweet wine made of the Concord grapes similar to those the Pilgrims found growing wild. But don't drink too much, or you'll also duplicate the three "wilde days" of celebrating in which the colonists and natives engaged.

This original Plymouth Thanksgiving dinner tallies but 869 calories. And, while it is a little high on carbohydrates, it is low in fat—both the saturated and unsaturated kinds. It also provides an ample amount of protein.

If you are a hunter and have some wild duck or venison in the freezer, it would be appropriate to roast and serve either or both with the fish. After all, Massasoit, the big chief of all Indians in that area, brought five freshly killed deer to the first feast.

Venison is a very lean meat. A dry 3½-ounce serving is only 126 calories. Basted with butter or salt pork and served with Cumberland or other wine sauce, it will score 150 calories.

Some of the Pilgrims bagged wild ducks for the feast. This meat is 138 calories per 3½ ounce serving. If you serve duck with its skin, the same portion will be 233 calories. Don't. Instead, add 50 calories for butter basting and sauce.

As for dessert, plum pudding or a berry dish would do well, both in the calorie and authenticity departments.

Plymouth Thanksgiving Dinner	
Cod or shad or venison or wild duck 3½ ounces	
Cornmeal bread (Johnny bread) 3 ounces	
Succotash 3½ ounces	
Beer 12 ounces	
Or wine (3 ounces)	
Plum pudding	
Total Calories	869

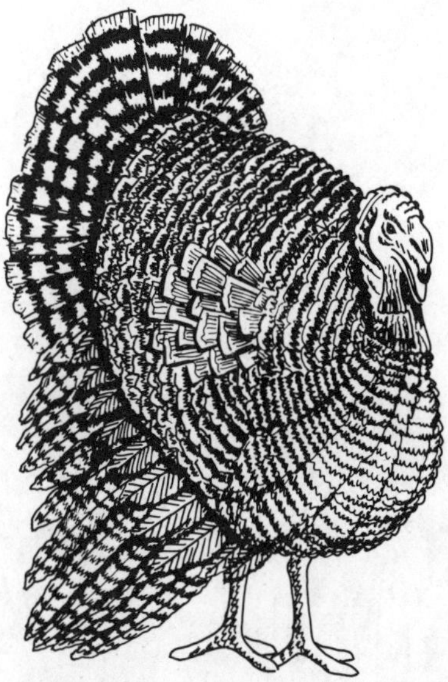

November — Week 4

Question: The favorite exercise of millions is jogging, walking, cycling, or swimming?

Answer: Walking.

Question: Which activity burns more calories over the distance of a mile—jogging or walking?

Answer: Neither burns more; they burn the same total number of calories.

Yep, more than 34 million Americans call themselves walkers. Walking is the number one athletic pursuit of Americans Canadians, Latin Americans, Europeans, Africans, Asians, Australians—just about everyone. And total calories come from the amount of effort expended. It takes one amount to go a mile; jogging is just faster.

Walking makes sense if you think about it. Your body is designed for walking. After all, that was how people got around before learning to ride on animals and in machines.

While we don't need to walk long distances to get places; we do need to walk to stay in shape. Look at the advantages:

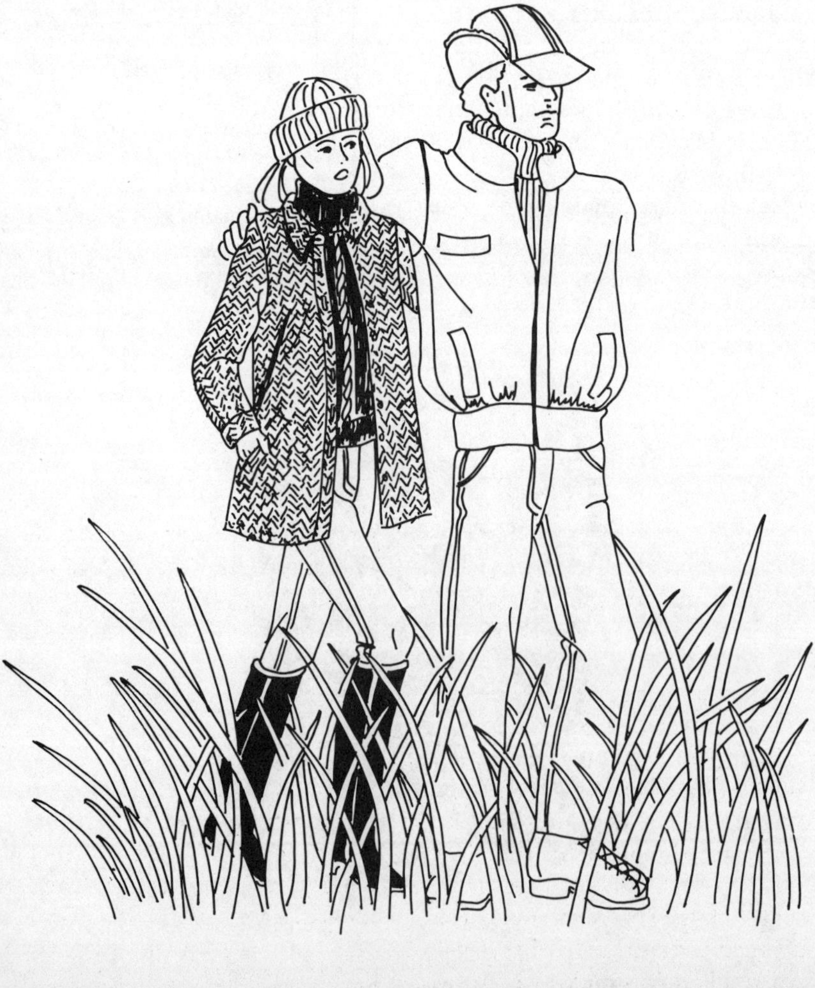

- You don't need equipment other than a good pair of shoes.
- You don't need special instructions or training.
- You don't need to be in peak shape to start.

In *The Complete Book of Walking* (Simon and Schuster, 1979), exercise expert Charles T. Kuntzleman and the editors of *Consumer Guide* tell how a mild walking program can take off 15 pounds a year, firm up your legs, and reduce anxiety and tension.

"Half an hour of vigorous striding burns 180 to 250 calories," Dr. Kuntzleman points out. That can add up to a yearly weight loss of 15 pounds Of course, if you eliminate some eating calories, you can multiply that loss.

Except for special instances, you don't even need medical clearance to start your walking program. Heart victims, arthritis sufferers, and even emphysemics can walk. And, unlike jogging, which imposes special stresses on the female body, both sexes can walk without fear of medical complications linked to anatomy.

Best of all, walking is an activity that you can do when you travel. Sure, you can pack your shoes and warmup suit in a separate bag if you jog, but walking in cities you visit is more convenient. Also, you will see more.

"One of the more enjoyable ways to get to know America—its people, customs, and cities—is to get out and walk," Kuntzleman wrote. To prove his point, the book offered walking tours, with maps of 24 cities from New York to Los Angeles.

Kuntzleman advises you to walk no matter the weather. But there are precautions to take: "High wind-chill factors are the greatest threat in cold weather, since you can get frostbite if you are inadequately protected from the wind. When you walk, your own motion against the wind increases the wind-chill factor and the risk of frostbite. Be sure that all normally exposed areas of your skin—head, face, ears, and hands—are covered.

"Dress in layers of clothing. This is very much like the insulation in your home: it keeps the heat in and the cold out. The layers of clothing trap warm air and hold it next to your body."

And by all means cover your head. It can release 80 percent of your body's heat. As one walker suggests, "If you want to keep your feet warm, wear a cap."

Dr. Kuntzleman has a schedule for getting you started on your walking program. Once you can do what the level requires, you move on to the next level.

Level 1: Walk 20 minutes a day 4 times a week, or 15 minutes a day 6 times a week.
Level 2: Walk 25 minutes a day 4 times a week, or 17 minutes a day 6 times a week.
Level 3: Walk 30 minutes a day 4 times a week, or 20 minutes a day 6 times a week.
Level 4: Walk 35 minutes a day 4 times a week, or 23 minutes a day 6 times a week.
Level 5: Walk 40 minutes a day 4 times a week, or 26 minutes a day 6 times a week.
Level 6: Walk 45 minutes a day 4 times a week, or 30 minutes a day 6 times a week.

Here's how-to-walk advice from Sandra Rosenzweig, in *Sportfitness for Women* (Harper & Row, 1982):

Walk briskly. Point your feet straight ahead. Put your heel down first, feeling your weight distribute itself evenly along the outside of your foot as you rock forward onto the ball of your foot and then your big toe. Stretch out with your stride and swing your arms in a natural rhythm with your feet, right arm forward as the left foot steps forward, left arm out as the right foot moves ahead. Slightly bend your arms and swing them loosely from the shoulders. Relax your hands so that your wrists flap slightly with each motion and your fingers are gently curled. Do not move your hands across your body. As you walk, hold your head high.

December — Week 1

You don't have to stop jogging in winter. But you do have to prepare yourself for the weather. That's the advice of Dr. Leonard Winston, a Chicago podiatrist who is himself a jogger.

If you want to continue outdoor running, snow is all right. In fact, it acts to cushion the impact of each step. (That impact is three times your body weight.) But there are precautions. Obviously, you can't run in knee-high snow. Nor should you allow your feet to get wet. Wetness is one of the major causes of blisters. They occur as a reaction to the irritation caused by socks rubbing against skin. When dry, socks and skin move together, and there is no rubbing.

So, if you choose to run in snow or on wet pavement, wear rubbers or galoshes over your jogging shoes. Or get a pair of rubberized, waterproof shoes. If they have cleats to grab the snow, all the better.

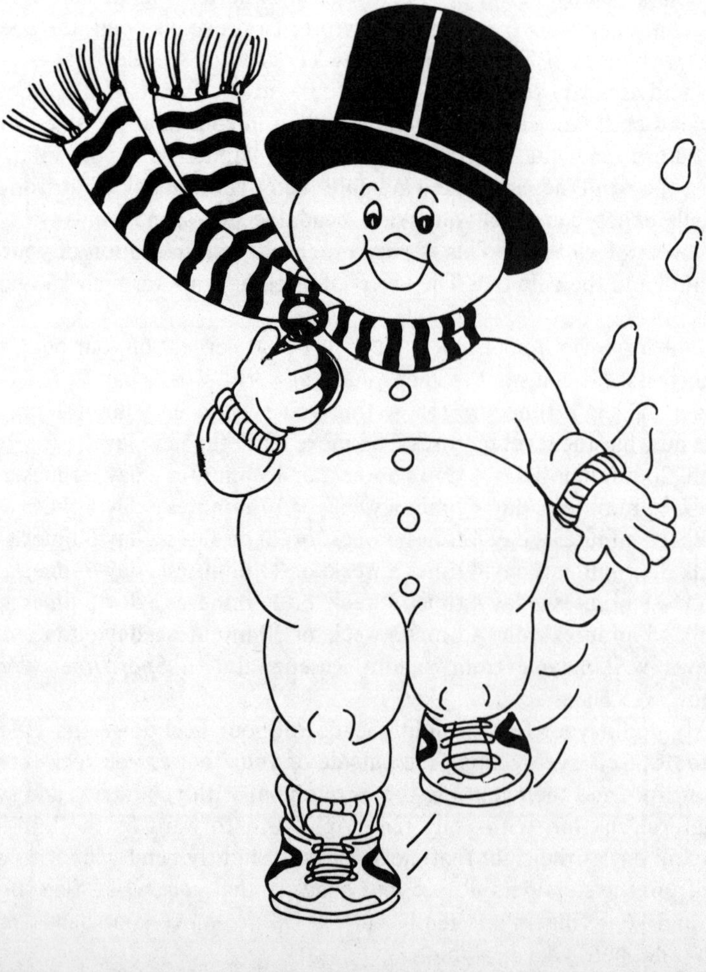

When the snow is high, or the pavement is icy or slippery, think twice. If you are a devoted runner, you are probably a very stubborn person. You hate to give up a day's run for any reason. Like the car commercial, you're driven. You must run. You feel logy if you don't run. But better a solid loginess than a broken bone.

You need to pay special attention to the skin of your feet, which tends to dry out in the winter. This dryness is caused by the drop in humidity of the air as it cools. If your feet get too dry they'll crack and bleed. So be sure you keep your feet well oiled with skin lotion to hold in the moisture.

After a run (or at any other time) give your feet a treat in the form of a contrast bath. Use two basins or buckets. Put a capful of bath oil in each, then pour warm water in one, cold water in the other. (Don't use epsom salt; it tends to dry the skin.) Place your feet in the warm bath for 3 minutes, then place them in the cold water. Alternate between the two. When you're done, dry your feet carefully and massage them as you apply lotion.

Your feet will perspire when you run, even though it is cold out. So wear sweat socks. And make sure they are cotton so that they will absorb the sweat. If you feel really cold when you start, wear two layers of socks. And make sure they're clean. You can get athlete's foot in December as well as in July.

Dress warmly, but not heavily. The best way to protect yourself against the cold is in layers of lighter clothing. This enables you to peel off clothes on the run as your metabolism increases and your body temperature rises. Expect to be warmer and to sweat more than usual because of the extra effort of running in snow.

In winter, a warmup is crucial. Never—but *never*—start running without doing stretching exercises. One of the best is to face a wall about a foot away, extend your arms, and lean forward on your hands. Then rock on your feet: up on your toes, then back on your heels. Each stretch should take about 20 seconds. Do a total of 2 or 3 minutes' worth.

Another good winter warmup: Standing, cross your ankles, balance yourself, and lean over to touch your fingers to the floor. It's OK if you can't touch; just trying helps.

These exercises loosen up the Achilles' tendons at the back of your ankles and the hamstrings at the back of your thighs. When too tight, these cause the most problems for runners.

Do the same stretching exercises after your run. Cooling down is just as important as warming up.

Of course, in winter you can also do your running indoors instead of out. You can run in place, run on a small trampoline, or run on a treadmill. A motorized treadmill that is sturdy enough for running costs $200 to $300. You can adjust its speed and incline to increase your work. A small trampoline will run $50 to $100.

Running in place needs no equipment. But there is a cost: some achiness at the beginning because you will be using different muscles than those you use in running distance. But after a week or so, these muscles will become used to their new job.

Best of all is an indoor track. Some Ys and community centers have them. Colleges and universities usually have hours when their indoor tracks are available to the community. Check it out.

December — Week 2

Your diet has never been in greater jeopardy.

Holidays are dangerous. Everywhere you turn there is food, food, food. The Hazardous Cs—cookies, candies, cakes—fill the landscape. A festive mood pervades every gathering of two or more persons. At work, at school, and at home you are urged to eat (after all, the word *festive* comes from "feast"). Work seems to be an activity sandwiched between parties these days. The whole world is baking or buying. Fat and jolly now go together. Almost everyone wants to be Santa Claus.

So, how does a dieter hold her or his own in what seems to be society's frontal attack on personal advances toward slimness? Here is some ammunition in the form of a dozen suggestions.

1. Keep your dieting to yourself. There are plenty of people out there eager to sabotage your efforts. You'd be surprised at how many of them are your closest friends and relatives. Holidays give them a renewed incentive to get you to eat.

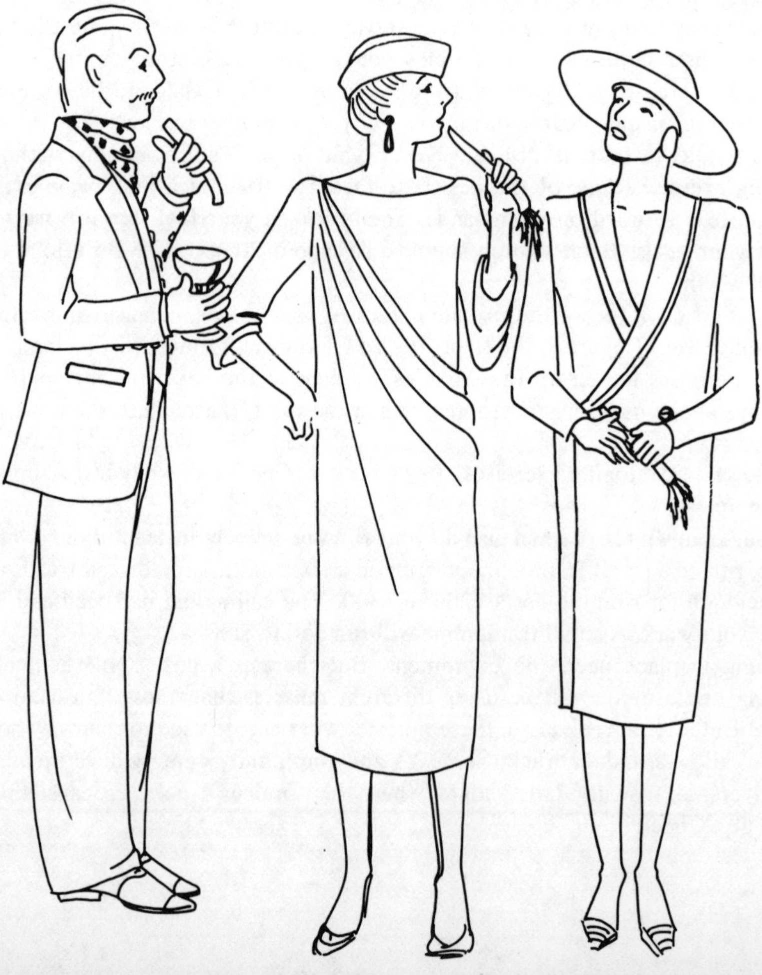

2. At the office, bring some diet snacks to counter the Hazardous Cs others put near the coffeepot. Put out carrot sticks, apple slices (sprinkle some cinnamon on them), and raw cauliflower pieces. (No dip, please.) By so doing, you're not preaching, you're merely providing an alternative for yourself and anyone else who cares to be careful.

3. In some circles, gifts of homemade Hazardous Cs are customary among friends. Start a new trend—give decorations or other handiwork of your own.

4. Before going to a party, always eat something at home. Arriving at a party ravenous will render you irrational and out of control. Since you plan to eat something at the party, don't eat a full meal at home. Try a bowl of soup and a few crackers.

5. Dress for the party in sexy clothes that are very form fitting, especially around your waist. That tightness will be a gentle reminder at the party to take it easy on the eating.

6. At the party, concentrate on the people, not on the food and drink. Your goal should be to meet and speak to everyone there, not to sample everything on the buffet.

7. As you circulate, stay as far away as possible from the end tables with their open dishes of "grab food" and from the buffet and from the bar and from waitresses serving hors d'oeuvres. When you decide to eat, make it a conscious decision. Carefully review all the foods on the buffet and select only what is on your diet. If someone notices you are not drinking and offers to get you one, ask for plain soda with a lemon twist or a spritzer of soda and white wine.

8. If you're afraid of offending your hostess, who keeps pushing food and telling you to sample this and that, parry her thrust by telling her, "Oh, yes, I haven't got to that dish yet. Thanks for telling me. It looks marvelous." Somehow you never get to it. An alternate parry: "Would you mind giving me the recipe?" She'll be so flattered she'll forget about keeping tabs on whether you ate the dish or not.

9. At a dinner party, pretend you are a diabetic vegetarian. That will keep you away from the foods that pack the highest calories—meats and their sauces and gooey desserts. If you know the hostess well enough, mention your food restrictions when you accept the invitation. Don't tell her you're trying to lose weight. That is a red flag, behavior that is not acceptable during the holidays. Tell her, instead, that your doctor allows you to eat only certain foods because of your "condition." You're not lying: Your condition is overweight, and your doctor has already told you to lose.

10. At informal coffee-and-dessert holiday get-togethers, drink plenty of coffee or tea and eat only fresh fruit. Stay away from the dessert table. Never eat standing up. One technique that works is to hold your coffee mug with both hands, or hold the saucer in one hand and the cup in the other. Politely decline offers of help to get dessert for you.

11. If you're giving the party, think low-calorie. Plan the presentation of the foods, since attractiveness is important. It will take effort, since most of us are taught to decorate cakes, cookies, and dip trays but not to arrange fresh vegetables or fruit decoratively on platters. As for the main course, keep it simple and forgo high-calorie sauces that include cream and flour.

12. Keep up your food diary and review it every night before you go to sleep. If you have been faithful to it, you will see where you have yielded to temptation and what you felt in those situations. This should help gird you for tomorrow's battles.

Above all, keep the joyous atmosphere of the holidays by getting high on people, not on food or drink. Use your mouth for talking, not for eating.

December — Week 3

During the Christmas season, you should take stock of what you have and what you would like to have. If you are in good health, consider that a major blessing. And if you are overweight, be thankful you are not even more overweight.

Be thankful for those around you who can and want to help. Perhaps you can suggest important gifts they can give that cannot be purchased in a store. (Give them this book to read.)

You don't want anyone to buy you a diet book—you'll buy the one you want when you want. Nor can anyone else buy your membership in TOPS or Diet Workshop or Weight Watchers or Diet Center or Overeaters Anonymous. If you are not now a member, you will join when you are ready. Lack of money is not what has been holding you back.

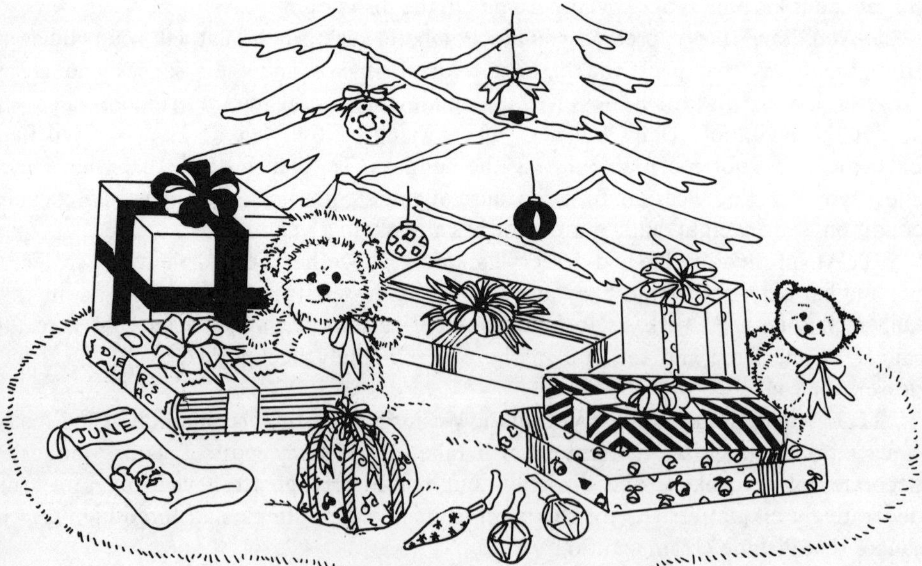

An important gift is tolerance. You need to be spared lectures on how terrible it is to be fat, how excess weight threatens your health, and how you would look so much nicer if only you lost some weight. You know all that.

Next is appreciation. You know you have a problem, and you need the support of the persons you love most. You need to feel important in their eyes. They cannot help you by criticizing your eating behavior or by withholding love from you because of that behavior.

You would be grateful if they withheld temptation. People who don't have weight problems often love to invite you out for coffee or ice cream, even though you have told them you would rather not. They are insensitive to the effects of environments polluted with temptations. Ice cream parlors are just one example; others are cafeterias, salad bars, convenience markets, and supermarkets. Other people's homes are also usually polluted with temptation in the form of munchies in open dishes on every table, and, in the suggestion of every hostess, "What can I get you?"

One of the best gifts you could get would be the understanding that you have chosen not to be overweight. People should realize that you are not happy with your body. Oh, it functions all right; it just doesn't look anything like those chic magazines say it should. You don't need anyone else's tsk-tsking to make you feel worse. Or more guilty. Somehow, you have been made to feel ashamed, as though being overweight is a sin or a crime. Rather, it is a bad habit. And only you can break that habit—only you, not your spouse or best friend or parents or well-meaning acquaintances.

The absence of false promises also would be welcome at this season of sincerity. You know, those promises made by every fad diet that comes along and by every new pill and diet food. Those close to you heighten the disappointment you eventually suffer by such touting as, "Have you heard about this great new diet? Ruth lost 10 pounds on it in a week"

A compliment is another great gift you yearn for. You'd feel much better about yourself if those close to you told you how nice your hair looks, or your clothes look, once in a while. It would be refreshing to know that their vision of you is not totally obscured by your fat.

Your loved ones could help immeasurably by not bribing you. You are probably too kind to point out to them what they are doing. It would be wonderful if somehow they realized that they, more than you, are using food as a weapon. When they feel good, or they want your favor, they take you out to dinner or provide yummy treats.

Bribery works in other ways too. Sometimes it is subtle, such as the promise of a trip to some sunny resort where you know lean, tanned bodies parade in bikinis. (So you'd better lose before you go.) Other times it is an outright bribe such as, "I'll buy you a fur coat if only you will lose 50 pounds." ($100 a pound!)

Bribes make you nervous. You know that one of the reasons for your compulsion to eat is nervousness. Others bite their nails or smoke; you nibble. Eating is your antinervous behavior. You will put food into your mouth much less often if those around you behave in ways that do not make you nervous.

The greatest gift of all is that of love, its substance and expression. You need warmth and affection. You need the assurance that you are loved and that the love is not related to any increase or decrease of fat on your body.

December — Week 4

As you face the New Year, face yourself.

Some people can lose weight, and what is more important, keep it off, by the force of their own will and solitary effort. But if you are like most dieters, you need fellow dieters to encourage and inspire you. Enter the diet group, an assemblage of persons like yourself, led by a dieter who has succeeded and who can pass along her secrets of success, along with the diet that helped her lose all those pounds.

There are lots of groups to choose from, especially in metropolitan areas, so take your time in choosing one for yourself. They range from businesses, like Weight Watchers International (WWI), to nonprofit organizations, like TOPS. Their approaches vary from WWI's slick yet effective package to Overeaters Anonymous's loose and in-depth approach.

You'll best serve yourself by shopping around and sitting in on sessions of the groups that most appeal to you. Any decision to join should be based on your experience, your feelings about the people who are in the group and who lead it, the convenience of meetings (time, date, location), and the cost (if any).

When making your decision, don't put too much weight on testimonials. There are avid proponents of every approach to weight loss. Every diet and every club has wrought its miracles. You are *not* looking for a miracle. You know that you can't click your heels three times and fly away to Slim Land. Instead, you want a group you feel comfortable with and with which you feel you can succeed.

You are likely to be struck by the observation that such groups are predominantly female. Here and there you'll find a male or two or three, but diet groups characteristi-

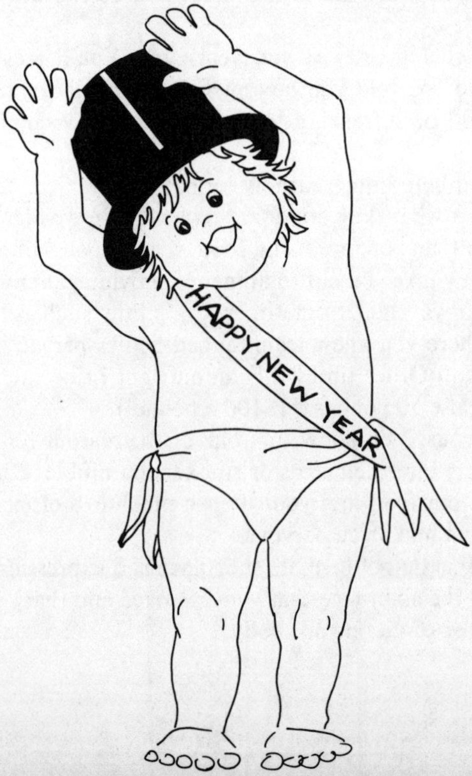

cally are female activities, with one exception: Sir Tops, the all-male TOPS group that meets at Skokie, Illinois, on Sunday mornings. Except for this club, diet groups present a female presence that you'll have to decide about.

There are many local groups as well as those of the big national and regional diet organizations. You'll find them all listed in your Yellow Pages under Reducing and Weight Control, or by name in the alphabetical section of the phone book. If you can't find its local listing, call or write the organization's headquarters and ask.

Here is a quick guide to the diet clubs. It doesn't include every one, just the major ones—major by size and geographical spread. Be sure you ask for rates. When you decide to join, make sure the rates are as quoted. Don't sign any contract without studying it and understanding it. And stay away from long-term or lifetime deals. You don't need them.

Again, each diet organization is different. The list here is in descending order of quality of program, diet, or both. Not listed are such physician-centered programs as NutriSystem and such nongroup commercial methods as Cambridge.

Weight Watchers International
800 Community Drive
Manhasset, NY 11030
Phone: (516) 627-9200
January 1983 marked WWI's twentieth year. During this time, more than 13 million dieters enrolled. The four-part plan includes diet, a behavior modification program known as the Personal Action Plan, the PepStep exercise plan, and weekly meetings. WWI also franchises summer camps for overweight kids and grown-ups, frozen foods, diet soda, and a monthly magazine.

The Diet Workshop
Suite 301
111 Washington Street
Brookline, MA 02146
Phone: (617) 739-2222
Not as huge as WWI, but as well organized and thought out, DW offers members a seven-cycle diet, an exercise program, and lots of personal attention. Private counseling sessions are also available. Unlike WWI, DW teaches you to count calories.

TOPS Club, Inc.
P.O. Box 07489
Milwaukee, WI 53207
Phone: (414) 482-4620
Oldest and largest of the diet organizations is the nonprofit TOPS (for Take Off Pounds Sensibly). In addition to helping its 336,000 members in 12,420 chapters in the United States, Canada, and 24 other countries, TOPS, a nonprofit charitable corporation, has contributed more than a $2 million to research into the causes and treatment of obesity, through a program headquartered at the Medical College of Wisconsin, also in Milwaukee. While it offers a diet, TOPS expects each member to consult a physician for diet and weight goals. Frankly patterned after Alcoholics Anonymous, TOPS emphasizes group discussion. Top losers are recognized at the annual convention.

Overeaters Anonymous
P.O. Box 92870
Los Angeles, CA 90009
Phone: (213) 320-7941
OA hews far closer to the Alcoholics Anonymous line than does TOPS. It offers no diet or dietary advice; instead, it focuses on compulsive overeating as a threefold disease akin to alcoholism and drug abuse, with physical, emotional, and spiritual components. Like other addictions, says OA, compulsive overeating can be arrested, but not cured. Also, while OA believes in the spiritual side of its program, it is not based on, or steeped in, religion. Nor is OA concerned with the medical and nutritional aspects of obesity.

Diet Control Centers, Inc.
1021 Stuyvesant Avenue
Union, NJ 07083
Phone: (201) 687-0007
With 250,000 members in New York, New Jersey, Pennsylvania, South Carolina, and Florida, DCC is modeled after Weight Watchers but offers more personalized services and a high-fiber, low-cost diet. Also offered are exercise and behavior modification programs.

Lean Line
151 New World Way
South Plainfield, NJ 07080
Phone: (201) 757-6446
Emphasizing low-calorie ethnic dishes (primarily Italian and Jewish), Lean Line has franchises in New York, New Jersey, Pennsylvania, Connecticut, and Texas. Behavior modification is also part of the Lean Line.

Diet Center
P.O. Box 160
Rexburg, ID 83440
Phone: (208) 356-9381
Claiming to be the "largest franchise company in the weight-loss industry," DC has 1,600 centers in the United States and Canada. More than 6,000 counselors meet daily with their dieters and supervise them on the DC diet. While this diet is adequate in most ways, it specifically excludes dairy foods so that a special DC supplement high in calcium and invert sugar is required.

Trims Clubs, Inc.
1307 South Killian Drive
Lake Park, FL 33403
Phone: (305) 842-9411
Trims considers itself more of an adult education service than a weight-reducing club. Its 50,000 members in 13 states (Illinois, Indiana, Wisconsin, Michigan, Ohio, Iowa, Minnesota, Pennsylvania, West Virginia, Tennessee, Florida, New Mexico, and California) are taught how to diet by following Trims' unique 21-day food plan, which "restores the chemical balance of the body."

SAMPLE OF WEIGHT WATCHERS NO CHOICE PLAN

DAY 1

MORNING MEAL

Broiled spiced orange	1 serving
Cereal	1 serving
Skim milk	½ serving
Beverage	

MIDDAY MEAL

Tomato juice	1 serving
Tuna salad	1 serving
Melba toast	1 serving
Skim milk	½ serving
Beverage	

EVENING MEAL

Roast turkey	3 ounces
Spinach	1 serving
Tossed salad with Herb vinaigrette dressing	1 serving
Bread	1 serving
Beverage	

PLANNED SNACKS

Fruit cocktail	1 serving
Yogurt	1 serving

DAY 2

MORNING MEAL

Grapefruit	1 serving
Cottage cheese	⅓ cup
Melba toast	1 serving
Skim milk	1 serving

MIDDAY MEAL

Cooked chicken	3 ounces
Carrot sticks with green bell Pepper strips	
Mayonnaise	1 serving
Bread	1 serving
Beverage	

EVENING MEAL

Stir-fried liver and vegetables	1 serving
Green salad with Vegetable oil plus vinegar and herbs	1 serving
Orange	1 serving
Beverage	

PLANNED SNACKS

Banana	1 serving
Skim milk	1 serving

DAY 3

MORNING MEAL

Tomato juice	1 serving
Scrambled egg	1 serving
Bread	1 serving
Skim milk	½ serving
Beverage	

MIDDAY MEAL

Vegetable	
Cottage cheese	1 serving
Melba toast	1 serving
Margarine	1 serving
Fruit cocktail	1 serving
Yogurt	1 serving
Beverage	

EVENING MEAL

Broiled sole	3 ounces
Green beans	1 serving
Tossed salad with Vegetable oil plus vinegar and herbs	1 serving
Beverage	

PLANNED SNACKS

Applesauce	½ cup
Skim milk	½ serving

THE DIET WORKSHOP CYCLE ZERO
600-CALORIE DIET

BREAKFAST
Egg
Whole wheat toast, ¼ slice
Orange, ½
or
Cottage cheese, 2T
Protein bread, toasted, 1 slice
Grapefruit, ½

LUNCH
Tuna, 3½ oz. can in water
Whole wheat bread, 1 slice
Berries, ½ cup
or
Cottage cheese, ½ cup
Melba rounds, 6
Cantaloupe, ¼

DINNER
Salad of leafy greens:
Dressing tomato juice, vinegar, lemon juice, herbs, and spices
Chicken (white meat), 4 oz. cooked, or Shellfish, 4 oz. cooked, or white-type fish, 4 oz. cooked
Carrots, 1 cup, or string beans, 1 cup, or zucchini, 1½ cup, or broccoli, 1 cup, or cauliflower, 1½ cup

BEVERAGES
Water
Tea
Coffee
Diet soda
Skim milk, ½ cup per day

EXTRAS
Mustard
Herbs and spices, all
Artifical sweetener
Salt and pepper
Vinegar
Lemons and limes
Pan spray

DIET CONTROL CENTERS' 7 DAY MENU

DAY 1

BREAKFAST
4 oz. orange juice
¾ cup dry cereal with 4 oz. skim milk
Beverage, sweetener if desired

LUNCH
Cottage Cheese Sundae (3-4 oz. cottage cheese, ½ cup pineapple chunks, sugar-free gelatin cubes, 1 tbsp. chopped nuts, chopped lettuce)
½ oz. crackers

SNACK
1 apple

DINNER
1 c. vegetarian bouillon
3-4 oz. veal, peppers, and onions
½ cup pasta
½ cup spaghetti sauce

SNACK
6 oz. sugar-free yogurt

DAY 2

BREAKFAST
½ cantaloupe
¾ cup oatmeal with brown sugar replacement
8 oz. skim milk

LUNCH
2 hard-cooked eggs
Tossed green salad
1 oz. corn muffin
2 tsp. diet margarine
½ cup applesauce

SNACK
Chocolate milkshake (8 oz. skim milk, chocolate flavoring; blend)

DINNER
Bloody Mary (1 oz. alcohol)
3-4 oz. London broil
½ cup carrots
½ cup spinach
Lettuce and tomato

SNACK
½ cup fresh grapes

DAY 3

BREAKFAST
½ grapefruit
2 oz. tuna
1 oz. English muffin

LUNCH
*Chicken Salad Supreme
sliced tomatoes, cucumbers, carrot curls,
1 oz. roll

SNACK
Combine 8 oz. skim milk with 4 oz. strawberry diet soda; blend

DINNER
1 c. bouillon
3-4 oz. shrimp, onion rings, mushrooms, snow peas, water chestnuts—may be stir-fried with 2 tsp. oil
Sprout salad

SNACK
Peach Brandy Delight *

DAY 4

BREAKFAST
1 tangerine
1 oz. bread
1 oz. cottage cheese
1 tsp. sugar-free jam

LUNCH
4 oz. tomato juice,
Neptune Florentine*,
1 slice thin bread, ½ oz.

SNACK
DCC Hi-Energy Slimmer*

DINNER
3-4 oz. baked ham
½ acorn squash
½ cup green beans
½ cup crushed pineapple

SNACK
4 oz. frozen dietary dessert

DAY 5

BREAKFAST
4 oz. orange juice
¾ c. dry cereal
½ banana
4 oz. skim milk

LUNCH
3-4 oz. hamburger
1½ oz. roll
1 tsp. ketchup
lettuce and tomato

SNACK
½ cup berries with 2 oz. yogurt topping

DINNER
4 oz. white wine
3-4 oz. chicken
1 baked potato
½ c. wax beans
½ cup marinated aspargus on lettuce

SNACK
½ cup sugar-free pudding

DAY 6

BREAKFAST
½ cup citrus fruits
French toast
(1 oz. bread, 1 egg, 1 oz. skim milk)
1 tsp. sugar-free jam

LUNCH
1 cup bouillon
1 oz. chicken roll
1 oz. Swiss cheese on 1 oz. rye bread
Celery and carrot sticks
1 fresh pear

SNACK
Combine 7 oz. skim milk with 1 tsp. instant coffee; blend

DINNER
3-4 oz. broiled haddock
1 broiled tomato
½ cup zucchini
Tossed green salad

SNACK
½ cup canned peaches
4 oz. yogurt

DAY 7

BREAKFAST
½ cantaloupe
1 egg fried in 1 tsp of butter
1 slice bacon
1 oz. bread

LUNCH
4 oz. clamato
3-4 oz. tuna or salmon
tossed green salad
2 tsp. diet salad dressing
1 oz. roll

SNACK
8 oz. yogurt

DINNER
4 oz. white wine
3-4 oz. roast turkey
½ cup wild rice
½ cup carrots
½ cup Brussels sprouts

SNACK
Baked apple with raisins

* Indicates recipes included

CHICKEN SALAD SUPREME

3-4 oz. cooked chicken, cubed
1 apple cored & cubed
1 stalk celery, chopped
2 tsp. imitation mayonnaise
Pinch curry powder
1 tbsp. chopped nuts (optional)
lettuce

1. Combine first five ingredients; chill.
2. Serve on lettuce with nuts as garnish.

Recipe = 3-4 oz. Class 1 protein
1 Fruit
2 Optional — List A

PEACH BRANDY DELIGHT

2 tbsp. unflavored gelatin
½ cup cold water
¾ cup boiling water
⅔ cup nonfat dry milk
2 packets nonnutritive sweetener
1 tbsp. imitation brandy flavoring
1 cup sugar-free peaches
6 ice cubes

1. Sprinkle gelatin over cold water in blender container and allow to soften.
2. Next, pour boiling water into blender container.
3. Cover and blend until gelatin is dissolved.
4. Add dry milk, sweetener, brandy flavoring and peaches.
5. Blend at low speed until well blended.
6. Add ice cubes, one at a time, and process at high speed until melted.
7. Chill and serve in individual dishes.

Recipe = 2 Milk selections 16 oz.
2 Fruit selections

NEPTUNE FLORENTINE

4 tsp. diet margarine
3 Tbsp. chopped onion
¼ tsp. garlic powder
1 cup canned tomatoes
1 cup chopped spinach (cooked)
6-8 oz. fish (cooked) cut in bite size pieces (scrod, flounder, sole, etc.)

1. Saute onion in diet margarine until tender.
2. Add other ingredients and simmer until thoroughly heated and flavors combined (about 5-10 minutes). Serves 2.

Recipe = 6-8 oz. Class 1 Protein
2 Optional — List A

DCC HI-ENERGY SLIMMER

8 oz. skim milk, cold

1	tbsp wheat germ
1	fresh peach or
½	cup canned sugar-free peaches or
½	banana, or
½	cup berries, etc.

1. Combine all ingredients in blender.
2. Blend for 30 seconds.
Recipe = 8 oz. Milk
½ oz. Grain selection
1 Fruit selection

LEAN LINE'S 7-DAY DIET

MONDAY

Breakfast	1 oz. bagel	83 calories	1 bread selection
	1 oz. canned salmon or lox	50	1 breakfast protein
	1 tsp. cream cheese	50	1 oil & condiment sel.
	½ grapefruit	65	vitamin C fruit sel.
	coffee or tea (black)		
Lunch	8 oz. skim milk	80	1 milk sel.
	2 oz. ham	130	lunch protein
	lettuce, tomato, cucumber	40	free vegetables
	2 tsp. salad dressing (low-cal)	60	1 oil & condiment sel.
Snack	4 oz. apple	75	fruit selection
Dinner	4 oz. chicken breast (baked or broiled)	154	dinner protein
	2 oz. sweet potato (baked)	56	vegetable sel.
	1 tsp. butter	50	1 oil & cond. sel.
	cauliflower	12 per oz.	
	1 oz. dinner roll	75	1 bread sel.
	1 tsp. butter	50 c	1 oil & con. sel.
Snack	8 oz. skim milk	80 c	1 milk selection

TUESDAY

Breakfast	1 oz. whole wheat toast	75 calories	1 bread selection
	1 oz. American cheese	100	breakfast protein
	1 strip broiled bacon	53	1 oil & condiment sel.
	4 oz. orange juice	55	vitamin C - fruit sel.
Lunch	1 oz. pita bread	70	1 bread seletion
	2 oz. grilled hamburger	120	lunch protein
	shredded lettuce,	5	free vegetables
	tomato	10	free vegetables
	2 tbsp. catsup	36	1 oil & condiment sel.
	8 oz. skim milk	80	1 milk selection
Dinner	4 oz. crab meat or salmon (canned or frozen)	116	dinner protein
	lemon juice (squeeze)		
	celery, cucumber, green pepper, mushrooms,	40	free vegetables
	6 oz. ear corn	75	vegetable sel.
	2 tsp. diet margarine	40	1 oil & condiment sel.
Snack	4 oz. yogurt (plain)	80	milk sel.

	onion bouillon (envelope)	8	free food
	carrots	10	
	celery	10	

WEDNESDAY

Breakfast	2 oz. cottage cheese	60	breakfast protein
	4 oz. canned pineapple (drained)	55	1 fruit sel.
	1 oz. waffle	116	1 bread sel.
Lunch	4 oz. water-packed tuna	144	lunch protein
	salad greens	20	free
	4 tsp. low-cal salad dressing	50	
	¾ oz. matzo	100	1 bread sel.
	8 oz. skim milk	80	1 milk sel.
Dinner	6 oz. broiled shrimp	200	dinner protein
	4 tsp. diet margarine	80	2 oil & condiment sel.
	spaghetti squash	50	free
	4 oz. tomato sauce	41	1 vegetable sel.
	2½ oz. frozen dietary dessert	80	1 milk selection
Snack	8 oz. orange	80	vitamin C

THURSDAY

Breakfast	1 oz. cheddar cheese	100	breakfast protein
	1 oz. rye bread	78	1 bread sel.
	4 oz. low-cal cranberry juice	50	fruit sel.
Lunch	4 oz. orange & grapefruit	58	fruit sel.
	4 oz. part skim ricotta	190	lunch protein
	lettuce	10	free
	8 oz. skim milk	80	milk sel.
Dinner	4 oz. white meat turkey	200	dinner protein
	4 oz. acorn squash (baked)	39	1 vegetable sel.
	green beans	20	free
	1 tbsp. almonds	50	1 oil & condiment sel.
	1 oz. cornbread	103	1 bread sel.
	1 tsp. butter	50	1 oil & condiment sel.
Snack	8 oz. low-cal hot chocolate	60-80	

FRIDAY

Breakfast	1 egg-scrambled	80	breakfast protein
	1 tsp. butter	50	1 oil & condiment sel.
	½ grapefruit	60	vitamin C
Lunch	4 oz. broiled shrimp	140	lunch protein
	2 tsp. imitation mayonnaise	35	oil

	celery	5	free
	2 oz. hard roll	80	2 bread sel.
	8 oz. skim milk	80	1 milk sel.
Snack	4 oz. pear	70	1 fruit sel.
Dinner	4 oz. cod fillet (bake or broil)	190	dinner protein
	4 oz. potato (bake)	92	1 vegetable sel.
	4 tsp. sour cream	35	oil
	4 oz. zucchini	20	free
Snack	frozen low-fat yogurt	80	1 milk selection

SATURDAY

Breakfast	4 oz. plain yogurt	80	1 milk sel.
	1 oz. wheat germ	103	breakfast protein
	4 oz. pear	70	fruit
Lunch	2 oz. cold cuts (ham)	135	lunch protein
	1 oz. rye bread	78	1 bread sel.
	mustard		free
Snack	raw carrots, celery, cucumbers	30	free
	dip - 4 tsp. sour cream	35	1 oil & condiment sel.
Dinner	3 oz. roast beef (baked)	210	dinner protein
	broccoli	(10 per oz.)	free vegetable
	8 oz. stewed tomatoes	50	1 vegetable sel.
	1 oz. roll	70	1 bread sel.
	1 tsp. butter	50	1 oil & condiment sel.
Snack	8 oz. strawberries	80	vitamin C
	8 oz. skim milk	80	1 milk sel.

SUNDAY

Breakfast	2 oz. farmer cheese	70	breakfast protein
	4 oz. apricots	35	1 fruit sel.
	1 oz. whole grain toast	70	1 bread sel.
Snack	8 oz. skim milk	80	1 milk seletion
Lunch	4 oz. turkey breast	200	lunch protein
	salad, lettuce, tomato	20	free
	5 olives	30	1 oil & condiment sel.
	4 tsp. low-cal dressing	50	1 oil & condiment sel.
Dinner	6 oz. baked/broiled chicken	200	dinner protein
	3 oz. noodles	110	1 bread sel.
	2 tsp. gravy	44	oil
	broccoli	(10 per oz.)	free
Snack	4 oz. plain yogurt	80 c	1 milk sel.
	8 oz. orange	80	vitamin C & fruit sel.

NUTRIENTS

Nutrients know no time of year. They are always needed. Nutrients are the raw materials your body uses in the countless chemical reactions of life. Some of these reactions go on all the time; others occur only as necessary. But the basic chemicals—about 50 of them—must always be there. They are supplied by the nutrients in your food.

Getting these nutrients into your body is the basic purpose of eating food. Cooking, spices, preparation, presentation, and serving are all ways of making food appealing so that it will be eaten. So are cultural and religious occasions, such as feasts. (Emotional reasons for eating are a perverted impetus to eating, often leading to overeating and weight gain.)

Your flesh grew and has been repaired with chemicals made from nutrients provided to your body. At first, nutrients were fed through the umbilical cord from your mother, then in breast or bottle milk, and finally in the food you eat. Thus, you are the recombined chemicals of food you have eaten all your life. It's both that simple and that complex.

There are four major kinds of nutrients that your body uses for energy or for building and replacing tissues and their protection:

1. Protein: from the flesh of animals, poultry, and fish; from egg white; from dairy products; and from nuts and grains
2. Carbohydrates: the sugars in fruit and the starches in bread, pastries, and everything else made with flour
3. Fat: from meat, oils, nuts and grains, and milk products
4. Alcohol: the fermented product of sugar

All four major nutrients, while distinct, are chemical cousins. Each has a similar "spine" of carbon atoms. This allows these substances to be chemically converted from one to the other in your body.

There are other nutrients in food that do not supply energy or building materials for growth or repair or protection, but are still necessary. These are the many minerals and vitamins involved in the chemical reactions in your body.

The first step toward breaking down food to nutrients is digestion. From mouth to colon, the food you eat is chewed, pummeled, torn, and mashed; then it is chemically macerated by acids and enzymes in the stomach and small and large intestines. Proteins are broken down to their components, amino acids. Starches are broken down to sugars. Oils and fats are suspended as tiny globules—in effect, homogenized. At various sites along the digestive tract, these chemical raw materials are absorbed into the bloodstream and carried off to "assembly plants" in the liver and other organs.

Of course, not everything you eat is a nutrient. For instance, saccharin, the artificial sweetener, has no nutritive value. Nor do drugs. Nor do cellulose and other fibrous substances so plentiful in vegetables. That's why celery is such a good diet snack—it provides bulk and chewiness with very few calories.

Here is a closer look at specific nutrients.

Protein

The single most important food ingredient you eat is protein. In fact, *protein* means "of the first importance" (from the Greek *protos*, for "first"). About 19 percent of your body weight is protein. This includes muscles, bones, blood, and skin. In fact, aside from water, there is more protein than any other ingredient in your body.

Proteins are the basic life chemicals. Every living cell has them and depends upon them. Among the most important proteins are protoplasm (the substance of cells), enzymes (the catalysts that make chemical reactions work in the body), and hemoglobin (the red chemical of blood).

Protein is an intricate combination of molecules made of amino acids. After you eat a source of protein, five things can happen to its amino acids. They may be (1) oxidized for energy, (2) used to create body proteins, (3) converted to carbohydrate, (4) transformed into fat, or (5) excreted. To form new protein, your body puts amino acids back together much as you put together the letters of the alphabet to form paragraphs.

Many lower forms of life can make all necessary amino acids from scratch. Human beings can make but a few. Of the 25 amino acids that form protein, you need to eat eight. Your body makes the others. But it cannot store amino acids from food in any appreciable amounts. So it does two things with them: uses them immediately or converts them to other chemicals. The immediate use of amino acids to make protein takes place in the cells of specific organs.

For instance, the liver takes what amino acids it needs for its own responsibility: to make the clear part of blood (plasma), as well as certain blood-clotting chemicals. Then it takes excess amino acids, strips the amino groups (which contain the nitrogen) from their carbon spines, and converts the carbon and oxygen and hydrogen that are left to glucose for immediate energy, or into glycogen or fat for stored energy.

The breakdown of protein (and some other substances) to glucose is called *gluconeogenesis.* This powerful process is of major importance for the functioning of the body because it supplies glucose even if no carbohydrates are consumed (as on certain diets). As a guide, you may want to note that 100 grams of protein can be converted to 58 grams of glucose. The liver also takes old protein from the body and breaks it apart for elimination, like so much biological junk.

Doctors use "nitrogen balance" as the measure of the body's use of protein, since nitrogen is the hallmark of protein (it is found only in protein). When your body excretes as much protein as it takes in, it is in *nitrogen equilibrium.* When you eat more protein than your body excretes, you are in *positive nitrogen balance.* When your body excretes more protein than you eat, you are in *negative nitrogen balance.*

In nitrogen equilibrium, you are eating enough protein to take care of the wear and tear of living. If you are pregnant, or you are building up your muscles, as in weight lifting, your body may be in positive nitrogen balance. If you are starving of protein, you'll be in negative nitrogen balance.

Protein comes in various qualities in foods. High-quality protein (such as in meat and fish) contains all eight of the amino acids your body requires from outside sources. Low-quality proteins (as in grains) do not have all of these amino acids in the proportions you need; they are incomplete. Your body can make protein only when all eight essential amino acids are present—and present in the necessary, unequal amounts. If even one or two of these are missing, or scant, your body cannot form the protein it needs. If one or two are in short supply, it can make only a small amount of protein. In fact, the usefulness of any protein in foods is limited by the one essential amino acid that is in lowest supply!

Carbohydrates

Americans consume a third to a half of their daily calories as carbohydrates. Carbohydrates are essentially a plant product, made by green plants, using sunshine, to store energy. Thus corn, wheat, potatoes, rice, carrots, cane, beets, and all fruits are loaded with carbohydrates.

Carbohydrates are so named because in the early days of biochemistry they were thought to be carbon combined loosely with water. Chemically, this means that the carbon spine has "arms" of hydrogen and oxygen. Water is hydrogen and oxygen (H_2O).

There are three classes of carbohydrates: simple sugars, or *monosaccharides*; *disaccharides*, like the sucrose in cane sugar; and complex sugars and starches, or *polysaccharides*. The simple sugar, glucose, is extremely important. Called blood sugar, it is the chief fuel in your body. Every kind of tissue needs to "burn" glucose. Without glucose, your brain and nervous system could not function. You could not see. You could not think. You could not move.

After you eat a starchy meal or a rich dessert, the sugar content of your blood immediately rises. There are lots of kinds of sugars, but all are converted to glucose. The common kind of sugar in food is *sucrose* (cane or beet sugar). If you've had milk or ice cream, its *lactose* will be converted to glucose and galactose. If you've had certain fruits, their *fructose* will be converted to glucose too. If you've had a lot of meat, fish, or poultry, then *ribose*, a sugar in nucleic acids, in the nucleus of cells will be converted to glucose.

Your body may use some of the glucose immediately; it requires a minimum of 180 grams (about 6 ounces) a day. The liver removes most unused glucose from the blood, which is why blood-sugar levels fall back to normal in but hours after a starchy meal. This process is under the control of the hormone *insulin*. In diabetics, who don't have enough insulin, the extra sugar in the blood may "spill" into the kidneys, where it is removed and excreted through urine. That's why the urine of uncontrolled diabetics is sweet. (Ancient physicians diagnosed diabetes by tasting urine.)

Diabetics can experience the same *ketosis* as do dieters who are on no-carbohydrate plans, only worse. This occurs when the body burns too much fat for energy (more than 650 calories per day) instead of sugar. Severe ketosis produces dangerous acidosis, which may result in coma and death.

The liver takes what glucose it has removed from the blood and converts it into *glycogen*, a starchlike substitute, which it stores. (Muscles do this too.) The liver and fat cells also convert unburned glucose to fat. Glycogen is the body's short-range form of stored energy. Between meals, if the blood-sugar level drops too low, the liver converts some glycogen in its supply to glucose, which is released into the bloodstream for immediate use by tissues of the body. Muscles also convert glycogen to get instant energy for work.

Fats

Weight for weight, fats and oils yield more energy, or calories (a measure of heat), than any other nutrient. Since fat is a concentrated form of energy (9 calories per gram), it is used for long-term storage of energy by the body. It also keeps the vitamins, especially A, D, E, and K, in a form that makes possible their absorption by the body. Membranes of cells in your body need fats to function. Also, your skin, naked as it is to air and water, must be covered with a layer of oil or it will dry. People who have trouble digesting fat, or who are on low-fat diets for one reason or another, often suffer from dry, flaky skin.

There are three fatty acids that your body cannot make. That means you must eat them in foods. They are *linoleic*, *linolenic*, and *arachidonic* fatty acids. You need small amounts each day. The first two are present in soft vegetable oils, but you get arachidonic only from animal fat.

When you burn fats, certain portions of the fat molecule, known as *ketone bodies*, are released, and if present in excess quantities, they are excreted in your urine. This occurs in people who are on weight-reducing or other diets that include no carbohydrates. *Ketosis*, the state of the body revealed by ketone bodies in urine, can be dangerous. This is one reason why many doctors are opposed to such weight-reducing diets as Stillman's and Atkins's.

Most of the fats in our foods are in the form known as *triglycerides*, made up of four or five fatty acids. Also, some foods (especially red meat, egg yolks, and some shellfish) contain *cholesterol*, a waxy kind of alcohol. It is not found in plants.

There is a controversy centering on cholesterol's role in heart disease. Cholesterol is a component of the rustlike deposits that build up inside artery walls. Then a clot or spasm can cut off the flow of blood. When the heart's arteries (the coronary arteries) are involved, heart attack can result. This "rust," known as *atheroma*, essentially is an accumulation of fat and cholesterol.

Men who have had heart attacks in many instances have blood with unusually high amounts of cholesterol. These men usually ate diets high in both cholesterol and *saturated fats* (those that are solid at room temperature). When these men were put on diets low in cholesterol and high in what are known as *polyunsaturated fats* (those that are liquid at room temperature, such as corn oil), their blood cholesterol levels often dropped.

The cholesterol controversy is complicated by the fact that everyone's body makes its own cholesterol. It is necessary for the membranes of cells and as a basic chemical of some hormones. However, reducing the amounts of saturated fats in the diet, and cutting down on such high-cholesterol foods as egg yolk, usually can substantially lower the amount of cholesterol in the blood.

Finally, one last fact about fat: It has taste. In fact, most of the flavors in food go with fat. That's why we butter our bread and potatoes and deep-fry anything to improve its flavor. So fat is hard to give up.

Alcohol

Alcohols are another kind of food made of carbon, hydrogen, and oxygen. They are akin to carbohydrates. In fact, the favorite kind, ethyl alcohol, is made by fermenting one kind of carbohydrate: sugar. Most of the alcohol you drink is "burned" as energy; it cannot be stored or otherwise used, although it can be excreted in urine and breath. Of course, before it burns up, it produces its effects on the nervous system, dulling your senses and otherwise sedating you.

Vitamins and Minerals

Your body, like any other chemical factory, needs minute amounts of incidental chemicals to keep its main reactions going. These are minerals and vitamins, which combine with the esential food chemicals to provide energy, to help build new tissue, and to make hormones and other essential body substances.

Minerals help repair and restore cells that wear out and die and are removed from the body. For instance, iron and copper help make new red blood cells; calcium is used for teeth and bones; phosphorus for bone, nerve fibers, and other cells. You need only very small amounts of each mineral every day; but you cannot do without any for very long.

Vitamins are neither burned for energy nor incorporated into the protein of living tissue. They are necessary in other ways: to keep the body's chemical processes working. They never bring attention to themselves, but work quietly and efficiently. Only when they are absent would you know it; your body would start to malfunction in many ways, even leading to serious diseases such as scurvy and rickets.

There are two classes of vitamins. Those stored in the body are called *fat soluble*. These are vitamins A, D, E, and K. In large amounts, these vitamins are toxic and dangerous. Eskimos, for instance, have learned not to eat the livers of polar bears because of the poisonous concentrations there of vitamin A.

You can't store *water-soluble* vitamins. These include all the B-complex vitamins and vitamin C. In general, you can't accumulate toxic amounts of these vitamins, as the body washes them out in the urine. (The exception is vitamin B-12).

The best insurance is to take a vitamin supplement pill every day. The brand name is not very important; buy at supermarket and drugstore sales. Health food faddists say that "natural" vitamins are better than synthetic vitamins. However, vitamins work not by magic but by chemistry. Moreover, you may notice that "natural vitamin" advocates use only words and logic but not scientific research to persuade us. And they charge a lot more for "natural vitamins" than for synthetic vitamins.

At the end of this chapter is a chart that explains vitamins and minerals.

U.S. RDAs
(Recommended Daily Allowances used in nutrition labeling of foods.)

Nutrient	Adults and Children Over 4 years of Age
protein	45 to 65 g
vitamin A	5000 I.U.
vitamin C	60.0 mg
thiamin (B-1)	1.5 mg
riboflavin (B-2)	1.7 mg
niacin (B-3)	20.0 mg
vitamin D	400 I.U.
vitamin E	30 I.U.
vitamin B-6	2.0 mg
folacin	0.4 mg
vitamin B-12	6 mcg
pantothenic acid	10.0 mg
biotin	0.3 mg
calcium	1000.0 mg
copper	2.0 mg
iron	18.0 mg
magnesium	400.0 mg
phosphorus	1000.0 mg
zinc	15.0 mg

Calories

Calories aren't nutrients, but the four major nutrients have them.

If that sounds like a riddle, the solution is simple: Proteins, carbohydrates, fats, and alcohol can be used by the body as fuel. They can be burned to keep life processes, which require energy, going. Of course, nothing in your body burns with the temperature of fire. Rather, it is a biological sort of burning at about only 100 degrees F, a bit higher than the temperature of your body, which the fever thermometer measures.

A calorie is the unit that defines the amount of heat that can raise the temperature of a kilogram of water (about a quart) by 1 degree C. This is a thousand times larger than the calorie unit used in nonfood heat measurements. That's why the food calorie is technically referred to as the kilocalorie (abbreviated kCal.). In other words, calories used to total up therms used by your heating system are different units than the calories you total up in your food.

The calories your body uses while at rest determine your *basal metabolic rate.* Abbreviated BMR, the basal metabolic rate measures the amount of oxygen used to produce heat and is related to the number of calories also used.

As you age, your body's activities slow, and your BMR goes down. At age 12, normal BMR is 50 calories per hour; at age 90, normal is 32. The average BMR of a normal man 25 to 50 years of age ranges from 37 to 40. BMR usually is expressed in relation to the normal figure—that is, it might be -25 percent or +25 percent.

Physical activity shoots up your metabolic rate far above the base level. How high depends on how strenuous the activity. Thinking produces a negligible rise in metabolic rate. Metabolism is stimulated by the thyroid hormone.

Your body is in energy-heat balance. Since *thermal* means heat, and *dynamic* refers to movement, this is *thermodynamic* balance. A body in thermodynamic balance burns up as many calories as it takes in. This isn't necessarily a day-by-day balance, but a weekly or monthly balance.

During weight gain, your body is thermodynamically off-balance. You eat more calories than you use. The unburned calories are converted to fat and deposited under the skin. To lose weight, you must burn more calories than you get, and take fat out of storage to make up the deficit.

One last item about calories. Proteins and carbohydrates are 4 calories per gram; fat is 9 calories per gram; and alcohol is 7 calories per gram, or about 100 calories in 1½ ounces (1 jigger) of 86-proof whiskey.

VITAMINS AND MINERALS

The vitamin and mineral needs of the human body are complex and confusing to most persons. This simplified guide should help. For each micronutrient (as vitamins and minerals are called) you can easily find the RDDA (Recommended Daily Dietary Allowance), best food sources, and the bodily functions in which that micronutrient is involved.

You need some micronutrients in such infinitesimal amounts that you'll get enough on any diet. Other micronutrients are included here because you may have heard about them, even though RDDA's are not established. For some of these the importance to bodily functions is not established, either. More detailed discussions appear in the published sources upon which this table is based.

FAT-SOLUBLE VITAMINS

Vitamin	RDDA	Best Sources:	Functions:
A	4000 I.U.(b)	Liver, sweet potatoes, carrots, spinach, cantaloupe, squash, broccoli, and dried apricots.	Maintains skin, mucous membranes, night vision, and, in children, growth.
D	200 I.U.	Sun on skin, fish-liver oils, sardines, salmon, milk, dairy products, and egg yolk.	Bone growth and health, prevents rickets in children and spongy bone (osteoperosis) in the aged. Perhaps involved in the health of teeth.
E	8 mg	Vegetable oils (especially cottonseed and soya), margarine; shortening.	Contributes to the health of red blood cells, muscles, stomach lining, testes. Also important in pregnancy. In very polluted air dose should be increased as much as 400 mg.
K	70-140 mcg	Green leafy vegetables; tomatoes. Also made by bacteria in colon.	Necessary for formation of blood-clotting factors.

WATER SOLUBLE VITAMINS

Vitamin	RDDA	Best sources:	Functions:
B-1	1 mg	Pork and ham, whole grains, enriched flour and bread, peas, beans, and liver.	Prevents beriberi. Involved in carbohydrate metabolism and health of nervous system.

C	60 mg	Broccoli, citrus; and other fruits and liver.	Prevents scurvy. Involved in the absorption of iron, folic acid, amino acid metabolism, collagen formation, scar tissue, healing, drug metabolism, synthesis of steroids in the body, and white blood cell functions. Perhaps fights the common cold, in doses up to 1000 mg. Higher doses necessary when under emotional stress, on birth control pills and by smokers.
B-2	1.2 mg	Liver, milk, beef, pork, chicken, broccoli, salmon, eggs, and cheese.	Involved in protein and energy metabolism. Protects skin, mouth, eye, eyelids, and mucous membranes, including genital tract. Higher doses needed while on birth control pills. Sometimes useful in treatment of migraine headaches and muscle cramps.
B-3 (Niacin)	13 mg	Enriched flour and bread, meat, poultry, fish, liver, whole grains, and peanut butter.	Prevents pellagra. Involved in energy reactions, tissue respiration, fat synthesis of the body, health of skin and mucous membranes, and mental health.
B-6	2 mg	Liver, pork, meat, whole-grain cereals, and vegetables.	Involved in amino acid and protein metabolism. Ensures health of skin, mucous membranes, muscles, and mental state. Necessary for child's growth. Higher doses needed on high-protein diet or while on birth control pills.
Folacin (M)	400 mcg	Green leafy vegetables, liver, kidney, and yeast.	Prevents anemia by working with B-12 and iron to make hemoglobin. Involved in amino acid metabolism and synthesis of nucleic acids, which are necessary for cell division.
B-12	3 mcg	Liver, kidney, heart, meat, fish, eggs, and milk. Not found in plant foods.	Prevents anemia by working with iron and folacin to make hemoglobin. Required for normal functioning of body cells, especially those of bone marrow, nervous system, and gastrointestinal tract.
Biotin (H)	100-200 mcg	Yeast, liver, kidney, meat, milk, egg yolk, grains, and some fruits. Raw egg whites contain avidin which prevents absorption of biotin by the body.	Involved in metabolism of fats and carbohydrates in the body. Prevents dandruff, scaly skin, and depression.

Pantothenic Acid (B-5)	4-7 mg	Liver, kidney, heart, eggs and meat.	Involved in production of enery from breakdown of carbohydrates, fats, and protein.
Inositol	Unknown	Liver, yeast, fruits, juices, and cereals.	Not completely established, although it seems to be involved in fat metabolism.
Choline	400-900 mg in av. daily diet adequate	Egg yolk, cereals and vegetables.	A fat emulsifier, it is important for healthy nervous system and is involved in the structure of cell membranes.
PABA	Unknown		Not completely established, but may help keep hair and skin healthy.
Lipoic Acid	Unknown		Not established in humans.
Carnitine	Unknown	Meat	Not completely established, but seems to be involved in fat transport in muscle cells.

MINERALS AND TRACE ELEMENTS

Mineral	RDDA	Best Sources:	Functions:
Calcium	800 mg	Milk, cheese, salmon, beans, broccoli, oranges, sweet potatoes, lettuce, and beans.	Essential for growth of bones in children, hardness and strength of bones and teeth in adults. With sodium and potassium, it promotes rhythmic beat of heart and controls actions of nerves and muscle: necessary for blood coagulation: helps control passage of fluids through cell walls.
Phosphorous	800 mg	Milk, cheese, meat, whole grains and soft drinks.	Important component of the body's basic energy substance, ATP, and of the genetic code in nucleoprotein. Works with calcium to make bones and teeth strong and hard; activates many of the B vitamins.
Magnesium	300 mg	Seeds, nuts, whole grains, milk, meat, fish, and eggs.	Necessary for transmission of impulses along nerves and for contraction of muscles. Activates certain enzyme systems involved in energy transfer.
Iron	18 mg	Liver, beans, meat, spinach, apricots, peas, prunes, chicken, and tomato juice.	Essential to hemoglobin, the red protein in blood cells, and muscle tissue.
Zinc	15 mg	Meat, liver, eggs, and oysters.	Necessary for essential enzymes, insulin, nucleic acids, wound healing, growth in children, and prostate function in men.
Iodine	150 mcg	Seafood and iodized salt.	Integral part of thyroid hormones, prevents goiter.

Copper	2.5 mg	Oysters, nuts, liver, kidney, corn oil margarine, dried legumes, and raisins.	Necessary for absorption of iron and its incorporation into hemoglobin. Prevents nervous system degeneration; helps lower cholesterol levels.
Manganese	2.5-5.0 mg	Nuts and whole grains.	Essential part of bone structure. Involved in energy enzyme systems. Necessary for growth and reproduction.
Fluoride	1.5-4.0 mg	Drinking water, fish, and dry legumes.	Prevents dental caries and strengthens bones.
Chromium	0.05-0.2 mg	Brewer's yeast, meat, cheese, and whole grains.	Helps maintain glucose metabolism by working with insulin.
Selenium	0.05-0.2 mg	Seafood, kidney, liver, and meat.	Works with vitamin E to fight oxidative damage to cells.
Molybdenum	0.15-0.5 mg	Meat, grains, and legumes.	Important to function of several enzyme systems.
Sodium	1100-3300 mg	Salt, cured meats, and vegetables.	Maintains normal balance of fluids between fluids and cells and controls passage of substances into and out of cells.
Potassium	1875-5625 mg	Bananas, citrus fruits.	Works with sodium to balance fluids and regulate heartbeat.
Chloride	1700-5100 mg	Salt	Involved in acid-alkali balance of blood. Necessary component of gastric juice.
Sulfur	Unknown	Protein foods.	As an integral part of amino acids, it helps make proteins, keep hair and nails healthy. Involved in bile production.
Cobalt	Unknown	Meat	Important part of vitamin B-12 molecule and therefore essential to red-cell function. Important for bone marrow, nervous system, and digestive system.

Nickel, vanadium, silicon, tin, arsenic, and cadmium are trace elements known to be important. Required amounts are so small as to be easily provided in normal nutrition.

a. The Recommended Daily Dietary Allowances used here are for a female, age 23-50 years, 120 pounds, not pregnant and not nursing. Women in those two situations, and men, require slightly higher amounts.

b. International Units

SOURCES: Recommended Daily Allowances (Washington D.C.: National Academy of Sciences, 1980). John Marks, The Vitamins in Health and Disease (London, J.& A. Churchill, 1968). Ethel Austin Martin, Nutrition in Action, (New York: Holt, Rinehart and Winston, 1971), and Earl Mindell, Earl Mindell's Vitamin Bible (New York: Warner Books, 1979).

NUTRITIVE VALUES OF THE EDIBLE PARTS OF FOODS

(Dashes (-) denote lack of reliable data for a constituent believed to be present in measurable amount)

Foods approximate measures, units, and weight (*edible part unless footnotes indicate otherwise*)		NUTRIENTS IN INDICATED QUANTITY					
DAIRY PRODUCTS (CHEESE, CREAM, MILK; RELATED PRODUCTS)		Grams	Food energy Calories	Protein Grams	Total Fat Grams	Fatty Acids Saturated Grams	Carbo-hydrate Grams
Cheese:							
Natural:							
Blue	1 oz	28	100	6	8	5.3	1
Camembert (3 wedges per 4-oz. container)	1 wedge	38	115	8	9	5.8	Trace
Cheddar:							
Cut pieces	1 oz	28	115	7	9	6.1	Trace
Shredded	1 cu in	17.2	70	4	6	3.7	Trace
Cottage (curd not pressed down):	1 cup	113	455	28	37	24.2	1
Creamed (cottage cheese, 4% fat):							
Large curd	1 cup	225	235	28	10	6.4	6
Small curd	1 cup	210	220	26	9	6.0	8
Low fat (2%)	1 cup	226	205	31	4	2.8	8
Low fat (1%)	1 cup	226	165	28	2	1.5	6
Uncreamed (cottage cheese dry curd, less than 1/2% fat)	1 cup	145	125	25	1	.4	3
Cream	1 oz	28	100	2	10	6.2	1
Mozzarella, made with-							
Whole milk	1 oz	28	90	6	7	4.4	1
Part skim milk	1 oz	28	80	8	5	3.1	1
Parmesan, grated:							
Cup, not pressed down	1 cup	100	455	42	30	19.1	4
Tablespoon	1 tbsp	5	25	2	2	1.0	Trace
Ounce	1 oz	28	130	12	9	5.4	1
Provolone	1 oz	28	100	7	8	4.8	1
Ricotta, made with-							
Whole milk	1 cup	246	430	28	32	20.4	7
Part skim milk	1 cup	246	340	28	19	12.1	13
Romano	1 oz	28	110	9	8	—	1
Swiss	1 oz	28	105	8	8	5.0	1
Pasteurized process cheese:							
American	1 oz	28	105	6	9	5.6	Trace
Swiss	1 oz	28	95	7	7	4.5	1
Pasteurized process cheese: food, American	1 oz	28	95	6	7	4.4	2
Pasteurized process cheese: spread, American	1 oz	28	82	5	6	3.8	2
Cream, sweet:							
Half-and-half (cream and milk)	1 cup	242	315	7	28	17.3	10
Light, coffee, or table	1 tbsp	15	20	Trace	2	1.1	1
Whipping, unwhipped (volume about double when whipped):							
Light	1 cup	239	700	5	74	46.2	7
	1 tbsp	15	45	Trace	5	2.9	Trace

		Grams	Food energy Calories	Protein Grams	Total Fat Grams	Fatty Acids Saturated Grams	Carbo-hydrate Grams
Heavy	1 cup	238	820	5	88	54.8	7
	1 tbsp	15	80	Trace	6	3.5	Trace
Whipped topping, (pressurized)	1 cup	60	155	2	13	8.3	7
	1 tbsp	3	10	Trace	1	.4	Trace
Cream, sour	1 cup	230	495	7	48	30.0	10
	1 tbsp	12	25	Trace	3	1.6	1
Cream products, imitation (made with vegetable fat):							
Sweet:							
Creamers:							
Liquid (frozen)	1 cup	245	335	2	24	22.8	28
	1 tbsp	15	20	Trace	1	1.4	2
Powdered	1 cup	94	515	5	33	30.6	52
	1 tsp	2	10	Trace	1	.7	1
Whipped topping:							
Frozen	1 cup	75	240	1	19	16.3	17
	1 tbsp	4	15	Trace	1	.9	1
Powdered, made with whole milk	1 cup	80	150	3	10	8.5	13
	1 tbsp	4	10	Trace	Trace	.4	1
Pressurized	1 cup	70	185	1	16	13.2	11
	1 tbsp	4	10	Trace	1	.8	1
Sour dressing (imitation sour cream) made with nonfat dry milk	1 cup	235	415	8	39	31.2	11
	1 tbsp	12	20	Trace	2	1.6	1
Milk:							
Fluid:							
Whole (3.3% fat)	1 cup	244	150	8	8	5.1	11
Lowfat (2%):							
No milk solids added	1 cup	244	120	8	5	2.9	12
Milk solids added:							
Label claim less than 10 g of protein per cup	1 cup	245	125	9	5	2.9	12
Label claim 10 or more grams of protein per cup (protein fortified)	1 cup	246	135	10	5	3.0	14
Lowfat (1%):							
No milk solids added	1 cup	244	100	8	3	1.6	12
Milk solids added:							
Label claim less than 10 g of protein per cup	1 cup	245	105	9	2	1.5	12
Label claim 10 or more grams of protein per cup (protein fortified)	1 cup	246	120	10	3	1.8	14
Nonfat (skim):							
No milk solids added	1 cup	245	85	8	Trace	.3	12
Milk solids added:							
Label claim less than 10 g of protein per cup	1 cup	245	90	9	1	0.4	12

Label claim 10 or more grams of protein per cup (protein fortified	1 cup	246	100	10	1	.4	14
Buttermilk	1 cup	245	100	8	2	1.3	12
Canned:							
Evaporated, unsweetened:							
Whole milk	1 cup	252	340	17	19	11.6	25
Skim milk	1 cup	255	200	19	1	.3	29
Sweetened, condensed	1 cup	306	980	24	27	16.8	166
Dried:							
Buttermilk	1 cup	120	465	41	7	4.3	59
Nonfat instant:							
Envelope, net wt., 3.2 oz[1]	envelope	91	325	32	1	.4	47
Cup[2]	1 cup	68	245	24	Trace	.3	35
Milk beverages:							
Chocolate milk (commercial):							
Regular	1 cup	250	210	8	8	5.3	26
Lowfat (2%)	1 cup	250	180	8	5	3.1	26
Lowfat (1%)	1 cup	250	160	8	3	1.5	26
Eggnog (commercial)	1 cup	254	340	10	19	11.3	34
Malted milk, home-prepared with 1 cup of whole milk and 2 to 3 heaping tsp of malted milk powder (about 3/4 oz):							
Chocolate	1 cup of milk plus 3/4 oz of powder	265	235	9	9	5.5	29
Natural	1 cup of milk plus 3/4 oz of powder	265	235	11	10	6.0	27
Shakes, thick:[3]							
Chocolate, container, net wt., 10.6 oz	container	300	355	9	8	5.0	63
Vanilla, container, net wt., 11 oz	container	313	350	12	9	5.9	56
Milk desserts, frozen:							
Ice cream:							
Regular (about 11% fat):							
Hardened	1/2 gal	1,064	2,155	38	115	71.3	254
	1 cup	133	270	5	14	8.9	32
	3-fl oz container	50	100	2	5	3.4	12
Soft serve (frozen custard)	1 cup	173	375	7	23	13.5	38
Rich (about 16% fat), hardened	1/2 gal	1,188	2,805	33	190	118.3	256
	1 cup	148	350	4	24	14.7	32
Ice milk:							
Hardened (about 4.3% fat)	1/2 gal	1,048	1,470	41	45	28.1	232
	1 cup	131	185	5	6	3.5	29
Soft serve (about 2.6% fat)	1 cup	175	225	8	5	2.9	38
Sherbet (about 2% fat)	1/2 gal	1,542	2,160	17	31	19.0	469
	1 cup	193	270	2	4	2.4	59

		Grams	Food energy Calories	Protein Grams	Total Fat Grams	Fatty Acids Saturated Grams	Carbo-hydrate Grams
Milk desserts, other:							
Custard, baked	1 cup	265	305	14	15	6.8	29
Puddings:							
From home recipe							
Starch base:							
Chocolate	1 cup	260	385	8	12	7.6	67
Vanilla (blancmange)	1 cup	255	285	9	10	6.2	41
Tapioca cream	1 cup	165	220	8	8	4.1	28
From mix (chocolate) and milk:							
Regular (cooked)	1 cup	260	320	9	8	4.3	59
Instant	1 cup	260	325	8	7	3.6	63
Yogurt:							
With added milk solids:							
Made with lowfat milk:							
Fruit-flavored	8 oz container	227	230	10	3	1.8	42
Plain	8 oz container	227	145	12	4	2.3	16
Made with nonfat milk	8 oz container	227	125	13	Trace	.3	17
Without added milk solids:							
Made with whole milk	8 oz container	227	140	8	7	4.8	11

EGGS

Eggs, large (24 oz per dozen):							
Raw:							
Whole, without shell	1 egg	50	80	6	6	1.7	1
White	1 white	33	15	3	Trace	0	Trace
Yolk	1 yolk	17	65	3	6	1.7	Trace
Cooked:							
Fried in butter	1 egg	46	85	5	6	2.4	1
Hard-cooked, shell removed	1 egg	50	80	6	6	1.7	1
Poached	1 egg	50	80	6	6	1.7	1
Scrambled (milk added) in butter. Also omelet.	1 egg	64	95	6	7	2.8	1

FATS, OILS; RELATED PRODUCTS

Butter:							
Regular (1 brick or 4 sticks per lb):							
Stick (1/2 cup)	1 stick	113	815	1	92	57.3	Trace
Tablespoon (about 1/8 stick)	1 tbsp	14	100	Trace	12	7.2	Trace
Pat (1 in square, 1/3 in high; 90 per lb)	1 pat	5	35	Trace	4	2.5	Trace
Whipped (6 sticks or two 8-oz containers per lb)							
Stick (1/2 cup)	1 stick	76	540	1	61	38.2	Trace
Tablespoon (about 1/8 stick)	1 tbsp	9	65	Trace	8	4.7	Trace
Pat (1 1/4 in square, 1/3 in high; 120 per lb)	1 pat	4	25	Trace	3	1.9	Trace
Fats, cooking (vegetable shortenings)	1 cup	200	1,770	0	200	48.8	0

	1 tbsp......	13	110	0	13	3.2	0
Lard	1 cup	205	1,850	0	205	81.0	0
	1 tbsp......	13	115	0	13	5.1	0
Margarine:							
Regular (1 brick or 4 sticks per lb):							
Stick (1/2 cup)	1 stick	113	815	1	92	16.7	Trace
Tablespoon (about 1/8 stick)	1 tbsp......	14	100	Trace	12	2.1	Trace
Pat (1 in square, 1/3 in high; 90 per lb)...............................	1 pat........	5	35	Trace	4	.7	Trace
Soft, two 8-oz containers per lb	container	227	1,635	1	184	32.5	Trace
Whipped (6 sticks per lb):							
Stick (1/2 cup)	1 stick	76	545	Trace	61	11.2	Trace
Tablespoon (about 1/8 stick)	1 tbsp......	9	70	Trace	8	1.4	Trace
Oils, salad or cooking:							
Corn	1 cup	218	1,925	0	218	27.7	0
	1 tbsp......	14	120	0	14	1.7	0
Olive	1 cup	216	1,910	0	216	30.7	0
	1 tbsp......	14	120	0	14	1.9	0
Peanut..	1 cup	216	1,910	0	216	37.4	0
	1 tbsp......	14	120	0	14	2.3	0
Safflower..................................	1 cup	218	1,925	0	218	20.5	0
	1 tbsp......	14	120	0	14	1.3	0
Soybean oil, hydrogenated (partially hardened)	1 cup	218	1,925	0	218	38.2	0
	1 tbsp......	14	120	0	14	2.0	0
Soybean-cottonseed oil blend, hydrogenated	1 cup	218	1,925	0	218	38.2	0
	1 tbsp......	14	120	0	14	2.4	0
Salad dressings:							
Commercial:							
Blue cheese:							
Regular	1 tbsp......	15	75	1	8	1.6	1
Low calorie (5 Cal per tsp)....	1 tbsp......	16	10	Trace	1	.5	1
French:							
Regular	1 tbsp......	16	65	Trace	6	1.1	3
Low calorie (5 Cal per tsp)....	1 tbsp......	16	15	Trace	1	.1	2
Italian:							
Regular	1 tbsp......	15	85	Trace	9	1.6	1
Low calorie (2 Cal per tsp)....	1 tbsp......	15	10	Trace	1	.1	Trace
Mayonnaise............................	1 tbsp......	14	100	Trace	11	2.0	Trace
Mayonnaise type:							
Regular	1 tbsp......	15	65	Trace	6	1.1	2
Low calorie (8 Cal per tsp)....	1 tbsp......	16	20	Trace	2	.4	2
Tartar sauce, regular.............	1 tbsp......	14	75	Trace	8	1.5	1
Thousand Island:							
Regular	1 tbsp......	16	80	Trace	8	1.4	2
Low calorie (10 Cal per tsp)..	1 tbsp......	15	25	Trace	2	.4	2
From home recipe:							
Cooked type[4]	1 tbsp......	16	25	1	2	.5	2

FISH, SHELLFISH, MEAT, POULTRY; RELATED PRODUCTS

Fish and shellfish:							
Bluefish, baked with butter or							

		Grams	Food energy Calories	Protein Grams	Total Fat Grams	Fatty Acids Saturated Grams	Carbo-hydrate Grams
margarine	3 oz	85	135	22	4	—	0
Clams:							
Raw, meat only	3 oz	85	65	11	1	—	2
Canned, solids and liquid	3 oz	85	45	7	1	0.2	2
Crabmeat (white or king), canned, not pressed down	1 cup	135	135	24	3	.6	1
Fish sticks, breaded, cooked, frozen (stick, 4 by 1 by 1/2 in)	1 fish stick or 1 oz	28	50	5	3	—	2
Haddock, breaded, fried[5]	3 oz	85	140	17	5	1.4	5
Ocean perch, breaded, fried[5]	1 fillet	85	195	16	11	2.7	6
Oysters, raw, meat only (13-19 medium Selects)	1 cup	240	160	20	4	1.3	8
Salmon, pink, canned, solids and liquid	3 oz	85	120	17	5	.9	0
Sardines, Altantic, canned in oil, drained solids	3 oz	85	175	20	9	3.0	0
Scallops, frozen, breaded, fried, reheated	6 scallops	90	175	16	8	—	9
Shad, baked with butter or margarine, bacon	3 oz	85	170	20	10	—	0
Shrimp:							
Canned meat	3 oz	85	100	21	1	.1	1
French fried[6]	3 oz	85	190	17	9	2.3	9
Tuna, canned in oil, drained solids	3 oz	85	170	24	7	1.7	0
Tuna salad[7]	1 cup	205	350	30	22	4.3	7
Meat and meat products:							
Bacon, (20 slices per lb, raw), broiled or fried, crisp	2 slices	15	85	4	8	2.5	Trace
Beef,[8] cooked:							
Cuts braised, simmered or pot roasted:							
Lean and fat (piece, 2 1/2 by 2 1/2 by 3/4 in)	3 oz	85	245	23	16	6.8	0
Lean only from item 162	2.5 oz	72	140	22	5	2.1	0
Ground beef, broiled:							
Lean with 10% fat	3 oz or patty 3 by 5/8 in	85	185	23	10	4.0	0
Lean with 21%	2.9 oz or patty 3 by 5/8 in	82	235	20	17	7.0	0
Roast, oven cooked, no liquid added:							
Relatively fat, such as rib:							
Lean and fat (2 pieces, 4 1/8 by 2 1/4 by 1/4 in)	3 oz	85	375	17	33	14.0	0
Lean only from item 166	1.8 oz	51	125	14	7	3.0	0
Relatively lean, such as heel							

of round:							
Lean and fat (2 pieces, 4 1/8 by 2 1/4 by 1/4 in)	3 oz	85	165	25	7	2.8	0
Lean only from item 168	2.8 oz	78	125	24	3	1.2	0
Steak:							
Relatively fat-sirloin, broiled:							
Lean and fat (piece, 2 1/2 by 2 1/2 by 3/4 in)	3 oz	85	330	20	27	11.3	0
Lean only from item 170	2.0 oz	56	115	18	4	1.8	0
Relatively lean-round, braised:							
Lean and fat (piece, 4 1/8 by 2 1/4 by 1/2 in)	3 oz	85	220	24	13	5.5	0
Lean only from item 172	2.4 oz	68	130	21	4	1.7	0
Beef, canned:							
Corned beef	3 oz	85	185	22	10	4.9	0
Corned beef hash	1 cup	220	400	19	25	11.9	24
Beef, dried, chipped	2 1/2-oz jar	71	145	24	4	2.1	0
Beef and vegetable stew	1 cup	245	220	16	11	4.9	15
Beef potpie (home recipe), baked[9] (piece, 1/3 of 9-in diam pie)	1 piece	210	515	21	30	7.9	39
Chili con carne with beans, canned	1 cup	255	340	19	16	7.5	31
Chop suey with beef and pork (home recipe)	1 cup	250	300	26	17	8.5	13
Heart, beef, lean, braised	3 oz	85	160	27	5	1.5	1
Lamb, cooked:							
Chop, rib (cut 3 per lb with bone), broiled:							
Lean and fat	3.1 oz	89	360	18	32	14.8	0
Lean only from item 182	2 oz	57	120	16	6	2.5	0
Leg, roasted:							
Lean and fat (2 pieces, 4 1/8 by 2 1/4 by 1/4 in)	3 oz	85	235	22	16	7.3	0
Lean only from item 184	2.5 oz	71	130	20	5	2.1	0
Shoulder, roasted:							
Lean and fat (3 pieces, 2 1/2 by 2 1/2 by 1/4 in)	3 oz	85	285	18	23	10.8	0
Lean only from item 186	2.3 oz	64	130	17	6	3.6	0
Liver, beef fried[10] (slice, 6 1/2 by 2 3/8 by 3/8 in)	3 oz	85	195	22	9	2.5	5
Pork, cured, cooked:							
Ham, light cure, lean and fat, roasted (2 pieces, 4 1/8 by 2 1/4 by 1/4 in)[11]	3 oz	85	245	18	19	6.8	0
Luncheon meat:							
Boiled ham, slice (8 per 8-oz pkg)	1 oz	28	65	5	5	1.7	0
Canned, spiced or unspiced:							
Slice, approx. 3 by 2 by 1/2 in	1 slice	60	175	9	15	5.4	1
Pork, fresh,[8] cooked:							
Chop, loin (cut 3 per lb with bone), broiled:							
Lean and fat	2.7 oz	78	305	19	25	8.9	0

		Grams	Food energy Calories	Protein Grams	Total Fat Grams	Fatty Acids Saturated Grams	Carbo-hydrate Grams
Lean only	2 oz	56	150	17	9	3.1	0
Roast, oven cooked, no liquid added:							
Lean and fat (piece, 2 1/2 by 2 1/2 by 3/4 in)	3 oz	85	310	21	24	8.7	0
Lean only	2.4 oz	68	175	20	10	3.5	0
Shoulder cut, simmered:							
Lean and fat (3 pieces, 2 1/2 by 2 1/2 by 1/4 in)	3 oz	85	320	20	26	9.3	0
Lean only from item 196	2.2 oz	63	135	18	6	2.2	0
Sausages (see also Luncheon meat (items 190-191)):							
Bologna, slice (8 per 8-oz pkg)	1 slice	28	85	3	8	3.0	Trace
Braunschweiger, slice (6 per 6-oz pkg)	1 slice	28	90	4	8	2.6	1
Brown and serve (10-11 per 8-oz pkg), browned	1 link	17	70	3	6	2.3	Trace
Deviled ham, canned	1 tbsp	13	45	2	4	1.5	0
Frankfurter (8 per 1-lb pkg), cooked (reheated)	1 frankfurter	56	170	7	15	5.6	1
Meat, potted (beef, chicken, turkey), canned	1 tbsp	13	30	2	2	—	0
Pork link (16 per 1-lb pkg), cooked	1 link	13	60	2	6	2.1	Trace
Salami:							
Dry type, slice (12 per 4-oz pkg)	1 slice	10	45	2	4	1.6	Trace
Cooked type, slice (8 per 8-oz pkg)	1 slice	28	90	6	7	3.1	Trace
Vienna sausage (7 per 4-oz can)	1 sausage	16	40	2	3	1.2	Trace
Veal, medium fat, cooked, bone removed:							
Cutlet (4 1/8 by 2 1/4 by 1/2 in), braised or broiled	3 oz	85	185	23	9	4.0	0
Rib (2 pieces, 4 1/8 by 2 1/4 by 1/4 in), roasted	3 oz	85	230	23	14	6.1	0
Poultry and poultry products:							
Chicken, cooked:							
Breast, fried,[12] bones removed, 1/2 breast (3.3 oz with bones)	2.8 oz	79	160	26	5	1.4	1
Drumstick, fried,[12] bones removed (2 oz with bones)	1.3 oz	38	90	12	4	1.1	Trace
Half broiler, broiled, bones removed (10.4 oz with bones)	6.2 oz	176	240	42	7	2.2	0
Chicken, canned, boneless	3 oz	85	170	18	10	3.2	0
Chicken a la king, cooked (home recipe)	1 cup	245	470	27	34	2.7	12
Chicken and noodles, cooked (home recipe)	1 cup	240	365	22	18	5.9	26

Chicken chow mein:							
Canned	1 cup	250	95	7	Trace	—	18
From home recipe	1 cup	250	255	31	10	2.4	10
Chicken potpie (home recipe), baked,[9] piece (1/3 or 9-in diam. pie)	1 piece	232	545	23	31	11.3	42
Turkey, roasted, flesh without skin:							
Dark meat, piece, 2 1/2 by 1 5/8 by 1/4 in	4 pieces	85	175	26	7	2.1	0
Light meat, piece, 4 by 2 by 1/4 in	2 pieces	85	150	28	3	.9	0
Light and dark meat:							
Chopped or diced	1 cup	140	265	44	9	2.5	0
Pieces (1 slice white meat, 4 by 2 by 1/4 in with 2 slices dark meat, 2 1/2 by 1 5/8 by 1/4 in)	3 pieces	85	160	27	5	1.5	0

FRUITS AND FRUIT PRODUCTS

Apples, raw, unpeeled, without cores:							
2 3/4-in diam. (about 3 per lb with cores)	1 apple	138	80	Trace	1	—	20
3 1/4 in diam. (about 2 per lb with cores)	1 apple	212	125	Trace	1	—	31
Applejuice, bottled or canned[13]	1 cup	248	120	Trace	Trace	—	30
Applesauce, canned:							
Sweetened	1 cup	255	230	1	Trace	—	61
Unsweetened	1 cup	244	100	Trace	Trace	—	26
Apricots:							
Raw, without pits (about 12 per lb with pits)	3 apricots	107	55	1	Trace	—	14
Canned in heavy sirup (halves and sirup)	1 cup	258	220	2	Trace	—	57
Dried:							
Uncooked (28 large or 37 medium halves per cup)	1 cup	130	340	7	1	—	86
Cooked, unsweetened, fruit and liquid	1 cup	250	215	4	1	—	54
Apricot nectar, canned	1 cup	251	145	1	Trace	—	37
Avocados, raw, whole, without skins and seeds:							
California, mid- and late-winter (with skin and seed, 3 1/8-in diam., wt, 10 oz)	1 avocado	216	370	5	37	5.5	13
Florida, late summer and fall (with skin and seed, 3 5/8-in diam., wt, 1 lb)	1 avocado	304	390	4	33	6.7	27
Banana without peel (about 2.6 per lb with peel)	1 banana	119	100	1	Trace	—	26

		Grams	Food energy Calories	Protein Grams	Total Fat Grams	Fatty Acids Saturated Grams	Carbo-hydrate Grams
Banana flakes	1 tbsp	6	20	Trace	Trace	—	5
Blackberries, raw	1 cup	144	85	2	1	—	19
Blueberries, raw	1 cup	145	90	1	1	—	22
Cherries:							
Sour (tart), red, pitted, canned, water pack	1 cup	244	105	2	Trace	—	26
Sweet, raw, without pits and stems	10 cherries	68	45	1	Trace	—	12
Cranberry juice cocktail, bottled, sweetened	1 cup	253	165	Trace	Trace	—	42
Cranberry sauce, sweetened, canned, strained	1 cup	277	405	Trace	1	—	104
Dates:							
Whole, without pits	10 dates	80	220	2	Trace	—	58
Chopped	1 cup	178	490	4	1	—	130
Fruit cocktail, canned, in heavy sirup	1 cup	255	195	1	Trace	—	50
Grapefruit:							
Raw, medium, 3 3/4-in diam. (about 1 lb 1 oz):							
Pink or red	1/2 grapefruit with peel[14]	241	50	1	Trace	—	13
White	1/2 grapefruit with peel[14]	241	45	1	Trace	—	12
Canned, sections with sirup	1 cup	254	180	2	Trace	—	45
Grapefruit juice:							
Raw, pink, red, or white	1 cup	246	95	1	Trace	—	23
Canned, white:							
Unsweetened	1 cup	247	100	1	Trace	—	24
Sweetened	1 cup	250	135	1	Trace	—	32
Frozen, concentrate, unsweetened:							
Undiluted, 6-fl oz can	1 can	207	300	4	1	—	72
Diluted with 3 parts water by volume	1 cup	247	100	1	Trace	—	24
Dehydrated crystals, prepared with water (1 lb yields about 1 gal)	1 cup	247	100	1	Trace	—	24
Grapes, European type (adherent skin), raw:							
Thompson Seedless	10 grapes	50	35	Trace	Trace	—	9

Tokay and Emperor, seeded types	10 grapes[16]	60	40	Trace	Trace	—	10
Grapejuice:							
Canned or bottled	1 cup	253	165	1	Trace	—	42
Frozen concentrate, sweetened:							
Undiluted, 6-fl oz can	1 can	216	395	1	Trace	—	100
Diluted with 3 parts water by volume	1 cup	250	135	1	Trace	—	33
Grape drink, canned	1 cup	250	135	Trace	Trace	—	35
Lemon, raw, size 165, without peel and seeds (about 4 per lb with peels and seeds)	1 lemon	74	20	1	Trace	—	6
Lemon juice:							
Raw	1 cup	244	60	1	Trace	—	20
Canned, or bottled, unsweetened	1 cup	244	55	1	Trace	—	19
Frozen, single strength, unsweetened, 6-fl oz can	1 can	183	40	1	Trace	—	13
Lemonade concentrate, frozen:							
Undiluted, 6-fl oz can	1 can	219	425	Trace	Trace	—	112
Diluted with 4 1/3 parts water by volume	1 cup	248	105	Trace	Trace	—	28
Limeade concentrate, frozen:							
Undiluted, 6-fl oz can	1 can	218	410	Trace	Trace	—	108
Diluted with 4 1/3 parts water by volume	1 cup	247	100	Trace	Trace	—	27
Limejuice:							
Raw	1 cup	246	65	1	Trace	—	22
Canned	1 cup	246	65	1	Trace	—	22
Muskmelons, raw, with rind, without seed cavity:							
Cantaloup, orange-fleshed (With rind and seed cavity, 5-in diam., 2 1/3 lb)	1/2 melon with rind[17]	477	80	2	Trace	—	20
Honeydew (with rind and seed cavity, 6 1/2-in diam., 5 1/4 lb)	1/10 melon with rind[17]	266	50	1	Trace	—	11
Oranges, all commercial varieties, raw:							
Whole, 2 5/8-in diam., without peel and seeds (about 2 1/2 per lb with peel and seeds)	1 orange	131	65	1	Trace	—	16
Sections without membranes	1 cup	180	90	2	Trace	—	22

		Grams	Food energy Calories	Protein Grams	Total Fat Grams	Fatty Acids Saturated Grams	Carbo-hydrate Grams
Orange juice:							
Raw, all varieties	1 cup	248	110	2	Trace	—	26
Canned, unsweetened	1 cup	249	120	2	Trace	—	28
Frozen concentrate:							
Undiluted, 6-fl oz can	1 can	213	360	5	Trace	—	87
Diluted with 3 parts water by volume	1 cup	249	120	2	Trace	—	29
Dehydrated crystals, prepared with water (1 lb yields about 1 gal)	1 cup	248	115	1	Trace	—	27
Orange and grapefruit juice:							
Frozen concentrate:							
Undiluted, 6-fl oz can	1 can	210	330	4	1	—	78
Diluted with 3 parts water by volume	1 cup	248	110	1	Trace	—	26
Papayas, raw, 1/2-in cubes	1 cup	140	55	1	Trace	—	14
Peaches:							
Raw:							
Whole, 2 1/2-in diam., peeled, pitted (about 4 per lb with peels and pits)...............	1 peach....	100	40	1	Trace	—	10
Sliced....................................	1 cup	170	65	1	Trace	—	16
Canned, yellow-fleshed, solids and liquid (halves or slices):							
Sirup pack	1 cup	256	200	1	Trace	—	51
Water pack	1 cup	244	75	1	Trace	—	20
Dried:							
Uncooked	1 cup	160	420	5	1	—	109
Cooked, unsweetened halves and juice	1 cup	250	250	205	3	1	54
Frozen, sliced, sweetened							
10-oz container	container	284	250	1	Trace	—	64
Cup	1 cup	250	220	1	Trace	—	57
Pears:							
Raw, with skin, cored:							
Bartlett, 2 1/2-in diam. (about 2 1/2 per lb with cores and stems......................	1 pear......	164	100	1	1	—	25
Bosc, 2 1/2-in diam. (about 3 per lb with cores and stems)..	1 pear......	141	85	1	1	—	22
D'Anjou, 3-in diam. (about 2 per lb with cores and stems)..	1 pear......	200	120	1	1	—	31
Canned, solids and liquid, sirup pack, heavy (halves or slices)	1 cup	255	195	1	1	—	50
Pineapple:							
Raw, diced	1 cup	155	80	1	Trace	—	21
Canned, heavy sirup pack, solids and liquid:							
Crushed, chunks, tidbits........	1 cup	255	190	1	Trace	—	49
Slices and liquid:							
Large....................................	1 slice; 2						

	1/4 tbsp liquid	105	80	Trace	Trace	—	20
Medium................................	1 slice; 1 1/4 tbsp liquid	58	45	Trace	Trace	—	11
Pineapple juice, unsweetened, canned..	1 cup	250	140	1	Trace	—	34
Plums:							
Raw, without pits:							
Japanese and hybrid (2 1/8-in diam., about 6 1/2 per lb with pits	1 plum	66	30	Trace	Trace	—	8
Prune-type (1 1/2-in diam., about 15 per lb with pits)......	1 plum	28	20	Trace	Trace	—	6
Canned, heavy sirup pack (Italian prunes), with pits and liquid:							
Cup	1 cup[18]	272	215	1	Trace	—	56
Portion	3 plums; 2 3/4 tbsp liquid[18]	140	110	1	Trace	—	29
Prunes, dried, "softenized," with pits:							
Uncooked	4 extra large or 5 large prunes[18] ..	49	110	1	Trace	—	29
Cooked, unsweetened, all sizes, fruit and liquid	1 cup[18]	250	255	2	1	—	67
Prune juice, canned or bottled..	1 cup	256	195	1	Trace	—	49
Raisins, seedless:							
Cup, not pressed down.............	1 cup	145	420	4	Trace	—	112
Packet, 1/2 oz (1 1/2 tbsp)	1 packet ..	14	40	Trace	Trace	—	11
Raspberries, red:							
Raw, capped, whole	1 cup	123	70	1	1	—	17
Frozen, sweetened, 10-oz container..................................	container	284	280	2	1	—	70
Rhubarb, cooked, added sugar:							
From raw	1 cup	270	380	1	Trace	—	97
From frozen, sweetened	1 cup	270	385	1	1	—	98
Strawberries:							
Raw, whole berries, capped	1 cup	149	55	1	1	—	13
Frozen, sweetened:							
Sliced, 10-oz container	container	284	310	1	1	—	79
Whole, 1-lb container (about1 3/4 cups).................	container	454	415	2	1	—	107
Tangerine, raw, 2 3/8-in diam., size 176, without peel (about 4 per lb with peels and seeds)	1 tangerine	86	40	1	Trace	—	10

		Grams	Food energy Calories	Protein Grams	Total Fat Grams	Fatty Acids Saturated Grams	Carbo-hydrate Grams
Tangerine juice, canned, sweetened	1 cup	249	125	1	Trace	—	30
Watermelon, raw, 4 by 8 in wedge with rind and seeds (1/16 of 32 2/3-lb melon, 10 by 16 in)	1 wedge with rind and seeds[19]	926	110	2	1	—	27
GRAIN PRODUCTS							
Bagel, 3-in diam.:							
Egg	1 bagel	55	165	6	2	0.5	28
Water	1 bagel	55	165	6	1	.2	30
Barley, pearled, light, uncooked	1 cup	200	700	16	2	.3	158
Biscuits, baking powder, 2-in diam. (enriched flour, vegetable shortening):							
From home recipe	1 biscuit	28	105	2	5	1.2	13
From mix	1 biscuit	28	90	2	3	.6	15
Breadcrumbs (enriched):[20]							
Dry, grated	1 cup	100	390	13	5	1.0	73
Soft See White bread (items 349-350).							
Breads:							
Boston brown bread, canned, slice, 3 1/4 by 1/2 in[20]	1 slice	45	95	2	1	.1	21
Cracked-wheat bread (3/4 enriched flour, 1/4 cracked wheat):[20]							
Loaf, 1 lb	1 loaf	454	1,195	39	10	2.2	236
Slice (18 per loaf)	1 slice	25	65	2	1	.1	13
French or vienna bread, enriched:[20]							
Loaf, 1 lb	1 loaf	454	1,315	41	14	3.2	251
Slice:							
French, (5 by 2 1/2 by 1 in)	1 slice	35	100	3	1	.2	19
Vienna (4 3/4/ by 4 by 1/2 in)	1 slice	25	75	2	1	.2	14
Italian bread, enriched:							
Loaf, 1 lb	1 loaf	454	1,250	41	4	.6	256
Slice, 4 1/2 by 3 1/4 by 3/4 in	1 slice	30	85	3	Trace	Trace	17
Raisin bread, enriched:[20]							
Loaf, 1 lb	1 loaf	454	1,190	30	13	3.0	243
Slice (18 per loaf)	1 slice	25	65	2	1	.2	13

Rye Bread:							
American, light (2/3 enriched wheat flour, 1/3 rye flour):							
Loaf, 1 lb	1 loaf	454	1,100	41	5	0.7	236
Slice (4 3/4 by 3 3/4 by 7/16 in)	1 slice	25	60	2	Trace	Trace	13
Pumpernickel (2/3 rye flour, 1/3 enriched wheat flour):							
Loaf, 1 lb	1 loaf	454	1,115	41	5	.7	241
Slice (5 by 4 by 3/8 in)	1 slice	32	80	3	Trace	.1	17
White bread, enriched:[20]							
Soft-crumb type:							
Loaf, 1 lb	1 loaf	454	1,225	39	15	3.4	229
Slice (18 per loaf)	1 slice	25	70	2	1	.2	13
Slice, toasted	1 slice	22	70	2	1	.2	13
Slice (22 per loaf)	1 slice	20	55	2	1	.2	10
Slice, toasted	1 slice	17	55	2	1	.2	10
Loaf, 1 1/2 lb	1 loaf	680	1,835	59	22	5.2	343
Slice (24 per loaf)	1 slice	28	75	2	1	.2	14
Sliced, toasted	1 slice	24	75	2	1	.2	14
Slice (28 per loaf)	1 slice	24	65	2	1	.2	12
Slice, toasted	1 slice	21	65	2	1	.2	12
Cubes	1 cup	30	80	3	1	.2	15
Crumbs	1 cup	45	120	4	1	.3	23
Firm-crumb type:							
Loaf, 1 lb	1 loaf	454	1,245	41	17	3.9	228
Slice (20 per loaf)	1 slice	23	65	2	1	.2	12
Slice, toasted	1 slice	20	65	2	1	.2	12
Loaf, 2 lb	1 loaf	907	2,495	82	34	7.7	455
Slice (34 per loaf)	1 slice	27	75	2	1	.2	14
Slice, toasted	1 slice	23	75	2	1	.2	14
Whole-wheat bread:							
Soft-crumb type:[20]							
Loaf, 1 lb	1 loaf	454	1,095	41	12	2.2	224
Slice (16 per loaf)	1 slice	28	65	3	1	.1	14
Slice, toasted	1 slice	24	65	3	1	.1	14
Firm-crumb type:[20]							
Loaf, 1 lb	1 loaf	454	1,100	48	14	2.5	216
Slice (18 per loaf)	1 slice	25	60	3	1	.1	12
Slice, toasted	1 slice	21	60	3	1	.1	12
Breakfast cereals:							
Hot type, cooked:							
Corn (hominy) grits, degermed:							
Enriched	1 cup	245	125	3	Trace	Trace	27
Unenriched	1 cup	245	125	3	Trace	Trace	27
Farina, quick-cooking, enriched	1 cup	245	105	3	Trace	Trace	22
Oatmeal or rolled oats	1 cup	240	130	5	2	.4	23
Wheat, rolled	1 cup	240	180	5	1	—	41
Wheat, whole-meal	1 cup	245	110	4	1	—	23
Ready-to-eat:							
Bran flakes (40%) bran, added sugar, salt, iron, vitamins	1 cup	35	105	4	1	—	28
Bran flakes with raisins, added sugar, salt, iron, vitamins	1 cup	50	145	4	1	—	40

		Grams	Food energy Calories	Protein Grams	Total Fat Grams	Fatty Acids Saturated Grams	Carbo-hydrate Grams
Corn flakes:							
Plain, added sugar, salt, iron, vitamins	1 cup	25	95	2	Trace	—	21
Sugar-coated, added salt, iron, vitamins	1 cup	40	155	2	Trace	—	37
Corn, puffed, plain, added sugar, salt, iron, vitamins	1 cup	20	80	2	1	—	16
Corn, shredded, added sugar, salt, iron, thiamin, niacin	1 cup	25	95	2	Trace	—	22
Oats, puffed, added sugar, salt, minerals, vitamins	1 cup	25	100	3	1	—	19
Rice, puffed:							
Plain, added iron, thiamin, niacin	1 cup	15	60	1	Trace	—	13
Presweetened, added salt, iron, vitamins	1 cup	28	115	1	0	—	26
Wheat flakes, added sugar, salt, iron, vitamins	1 cup	30	105	3	Trace	—	24
Wheat, puffed:							
Plain, added iron, thiamin, niacin	1 cup	15	55	2	Trace	—	12
Presweetened, added salt, iron, vitamins	1 cup	38	140	3	Trace	—	33
Wheat, shredded, plain	1 oblong biscuit or 1/2 cup spoon-size-biscuits	25	90	2	1	—	20
Wheat germ, without salt and sugar, toasted	1 tbsp	6	25	2	1	—	3
Buckwheat flour, light, sifted	1 cup	98	340	6	1	0.2	78
Bulgur, canned, seasoned	1 cup	135	245	8	4	—	44
Cakes made from cake mixes with enriched flour:[22]							
Angelfood:							
Whole cake (9 3/4-in diam. tube cake)	1 cake	635	1,645	36	1	—	377
Piece, 1/12 of cake	1 piece	53	135	3	Trace	—	32
Coffeecake:							
Whole cake (7 3/4 by 5 5/8 by 1 1/4 in)	1 cake	430	1,385	27	41	11.7	225
Piece, 1/6 of cake	1 piece	72	230	5	7	2.0	38
Cupcakes, made with egg, milk, 2 1/2 in diam.:							
Without icing	1 cupcake	25	90	1	3	.8	14
With chocolate icing	1 cupcake	36	130	2	5	2.0	21
Devil's food with chocolate icing:							
Whole, 2 layer cake (8- or 9-in diam.)	1 cake	1,107	3,755	49	136	50.0	645
Piece, 1/16 of cake	1 piece	69	235	3	8	3.1	40
Cupcake, 2 1/2-in diam	1 cupcake	35	120	2	4	1.6	20
Gingerbread:							

Whole cake (8-in square)	1 cake......	570	1,575	18	39	9.7	291
Piece, 1/9 of cake	1 piece	63	175	2	4	1.1	32
White, 2 layer with chocolate icing:							
Whole cake (8- or 9-in diam.)	1 cake......	1,140	4,000	44	122	48.2	716
Piece, 1/16 of cake	1 piece	71	250	3	8	3.0	45
Yellow, 2 layer with chocolate icing:							
Whole cake (8- or 9-in diam.)	1 cake......	1,108	3,735	45	125	47.8	638
Piece, 1/16 of cake	1 piece	69	235	3	8	3.0	40
Cakes made from home recipes using enriched flour:							
Boston cream pie with custard filling:							
Whole cake (8-in diam.)	1 cake......	825	2,490	41	78	23.0	412
Piece, 1/12 of cake	1 piece	69	210	3	6	1.9	34
Fruitcake, dark:							
Loaf, 1-lb (7 1/2 by 2 by 1 1/2 in)..................................	1 loaf	454	1,720	22	69	14.4	271
Slice, 1/30 of loaf	1 slice......	15	55	1	2	.5	9
Plain, sheet cake:							
Without icing:							
Whole cake (9-in square)	1 cake......	777	2,830	35	108	29.5	434
Piece, 1/9 of cake	1 piece	86	315	4	12	3.3	48
With uncooked white icing:							
Whole cake (9-in square)	1 cake......	1,096	4,020	37	129	42.2	694
Piece, 1/9 of cake	1 piece	121	445	4	14	4.7	77
Pound:[23]							
Loaf, 8 1/2 by 3 1/2 by 3 1/4 in	1 loaf	565	2,725	31	170	42.9	273
Slice, 1/17 of loaf	1 slice......	33	160	2	10	2.5	16
Spongecake:							
Whole cake (9 3/4-in diam. tube cake)	1 cake......	790	2,345	60	45	13.1	427
Piece, 1/12 of cake	1 piece	66	195	5	4	1.1	36
Cookies made with enriched flour:[24] [25]							
Brownies with nuts:							
Home-prepared, 1 3/4 by 1 3/4 by 7/8 in:							
From home recipe.................	1 brownie	20	95	1	6	1.5	10
From commercial recipe........	1 brownie	20	85	1	4	.9	13
Frozen, with chocolate icing,[26] 1 1/2 by 1 3/4 by 7/8 in	1 brownie	25	105	1	5	2.0	15
Chocolate chip:							
Commercial, 2 1/4-in diam., 3/8 in thick..........................	4 cookies	42	200	2	9	2.8	29
From home recipe, 2 1/3-in diam.	4 cookies	40	205	2	12	3.5	24
Fig bars, square (1 5/8 by 1 5/8 by 3/8 in) or rectangular (1 1/2 by 1 3/4 by 1/2 in)	4 cookies	56	200	2	3	.8	42
Gingersnaps, 2-in diam., 1/4 in thick	4 cookies	28	90	2	2	.7	22
Macaroons, 2 3/4-in diam., 1/4 in thick	2 cookies	38	180	2	9	—	25

		Grams	Food energy Calories	Protein Grams	Total Fat Grams	Fatty Acids Saturated Grams	Carbo-hydrate Grams
Oatmeal with raisins, 2 5/8-in diam., 1/4 in thick	4 cookies	52	235	3	8	2.0	38
Plain, prepared from commercial chilled dough, 2 1/2-in diam., 1/4 in thick	4 cookies	48	240	2	12	3.0	31
Sandwich type (chocolate or vanilla), 1 3/4-in diam., 3/8 in thick	4 cookies	40	200	2	9	2.2	28
Vanilla wafers, 1 3/4-in diam., 1/4 in thick.	10 cookies	40	185	2	6	—	30
Cornmeal:							
Whole-ground, unbolted, dry form	1 cup	122	435	11	5	.5	90
Bolted (nearly whole-grain), dry form	1 cup	122	440	11	4	.5	91
Degermed, enriched:							
Dry form	1 cup	138	500	11	2	.2	108
Cooked	1 cup	240	120	3	Trace	Trace	26
Degermed, unenriched:							
Dry form	1 cup	138	500	11	2	.2	108
Cooked	1 cup	240	120	3	Trace	Trace	26
Crackers:[20]							
Graham, plain, 2 1/2-in square	2 crackers	14	55	1	1	.3	10
Rye wafers, whole-grain, 1 7/8 by 3 1/2 in	2 wafers	13	45	2	Trace	—	10
Saltines, made with enriched flour	4 crackers or 1 packet	11	50	1	1	.3	8
Danish pastry (enriched flour), plain without fruit or nuts:[27]							
Packaged ring, 12 oz	1 ring	340	1,435	25	80	24.3	155
Round piece, about 4 1/4-in diam. by 1 in.	1 pastry	65	275	5	15	4.7	30
Ounce	1 oz	28	120	2	7	2.0	13
Doughnuts, made with enriched flour:[21]							
Cake type, plain, 2 1/2-in diam., 1 in high	1 doughnut	25	100	1	5	1.2	13
Yeast-leavened, glazed 3 3/4-in diam., 1 1/4 in high	1 doughnut	50	205	3	11	3.3	22
Macaroni, enriched, cooked (cut lengths, elbows, shells):							
Firm stage (hot)	1 cup	130	190	7	1	—	39
Tender stage:							
Cold macaroni	1 cup	105	115	4	Trace	—	24
Hot macaroni	1 cup	140	155	5	1	—	32

Macaroni (enriched) and cheese:							
Canned[28]	1 cup	240	230	9	10	4.2	26
From home recipe (served hot)[29]	1 cup	200	430	17	22	8.9	40
Muffins made with enriched flour:[20]							
From home recipe:							
Blueberry, 2 3/8-in diam., 1 1/2 in high	1 muffin	40	110	3	4	1.1	17
Bran	1 muffin	40	105	3	4	1.2	17
Corn (enriched degermed cornmeal and flour), 2 3/8-in diam., 1 1/2 in high	1 muffin	40	125	3	4	1.2	19
Plain, 3-in diam., 1 1/2 in high	1 muffin	40	120	3	4	1.0	17
From mix, egg, milk:							
Corn, 2 3/8-in diam., 1 1/2 in high[30]	1 muffin	40	130	3	4	1.2	20
Noodles (egg noodles), enriched, cooked	1 cup	160	200	7	2	—	37
Noodles, chow mein, canned	1 cup	45	220	6	11	—	26
Pancakes, (4-in diam.):[20]							
Buckwheat, made from mix (with buckwheat and enriched flours), egg and milk added	1 cake	27	55	2	2	.8	6
Plain:							
Made from home recipe using enriched flour	1 cake	27	60	2	2	.5	9
Made from mix with enriched flour, egg and milk added	1 cake	27	60	2	2	.7	9
Pies, piecrust made with enriched flour, vegetable shortening (9-in diam.):							
Apple:							
Whole	1 pie	945	2,240	21	105	27.0	360
Sector, 1/7 of pie	1 sector	135	345	3	15	3.9	51
Banana cream:							
Whole	1 pie	910	2,010	41	85	26.7	279
Sector, 1/7 of pie	1 sector	130	285	6	12	3.8	40
Blueberry:							
Whole	1 pie	945	2,285	23	102	24.8	330
Sector, 1/7 of pie	1 sector	135	325	3	15	3.5	47
Cherry:							
Whole	1 pie	945	2,465	25	107	28.2	363
Sector, 1/7 of pie	1 sector	135	350	4	15	4.0	52
Custard:							
Whole	1 pie	910	1,985	56	101	33.9	213
Sector, 1/7 of pie	1 sector	130	285	8	14	4.8	30
Lemon meringue:							
Whole	1 pie	840	2,140	31	86	26.1	317
Sector, 1/7 of pie	1 sector	120	305	4	12	3.7	45
Mince:							

		Grams	Food energy Calories	Protein Grams	Total Fat Grams	Fatty Acids Saturated Grams	Carbo-hydrate Grams
Whole	1 pie	945	2,560	24	109	28.0	389
Sector, 1/7 of pie	1 sector	135	365	3	16	4.0	56
Peach:							
Whole	1 pie	945	2,410	24	101	24.8	361
Sector, 1/7 of pie	1 sector	135	345	3	14	3.5	52
Pecan:							
Whole	1 pie	825	3,450	42	189	27.8	423
Sector, 1/7 of pie	1 sector	118	495	6	27	4.0	61
Pumpkin:							
Whole	1 pie	910	1,920	36	102	37.4	223
Sector, 1/7 of pie	1 sector	130	275	5	15	5.4	32
Piecrust (home recipe) made with enriched flour and vegetable shortening, baked	1 pie shell, 9-in diam	180	900	11	60	14.8	79
Piecrust mix with enriched flour and vegetable shortening, 10-oz pkg. prepared and baked	Piecrust for 2-crust pie, 9-in diam	320	1,485	20	93	22.7	141
Pizza (cheese) baked, 4 3/4-in sector; 1/8 of 12-in diam. pie[9]	1 sector	60	145	6	4	1.7	22
Popcorn, popped:							
Plain, large kernel	1 cup	6	25	1	Trace	Trace	5
With oil (coconut) and salt added, large kernel	1 cup	9	40	1	2	1.5	5
Sugar coated	1 cup	35	135	2	1	.5	30
Pretzels, made with enriched flour:							
Dutch twisted, 2 3/4 by 2 5/8 in	1 pretzel	16	60	2	1	—	12
Thin, twisted, 3 1/4 by 2 1/4 by 1/4 in	10 pretzels	60	235	6	3	—	46
Stick, 2 1/4 in long	10 pretzels	3	10	Trace	Trace	—	2
Rice, white, enriched:							
Instant, ready-to-serve, hot	1 cup	165	180	4	Trace	Trace	40
Long grain:							
Raw	1 cup	185	670	12	1	.2	149
Cooked, served hot	1 cup	205	225	4	Trace	.1	50
Parboiled:							
Raw	1 cup	185	685	14	1	.2	150
Cooked, served hot	1 cup	175	185	4	Trace	.1	41
Rolls, enriched:[20]							
Commercial:							

Brown-and-serve (12 per 12-oz pkg), browned.............	1 roll	26	85	2	2	.4	14
Cloverleaf or pan, 2 1/2-in diam., 2 in high.....................	1 roll	28	85	2	2	.4	15
Frankfurter and hamburger (8 per 11 1/2-oz pkg)	1 roll	40	120	3	2	.5	21
Hard, 3 3/4-in diam., 2 in high......................................	1 roll	50	155	5	2	.4	30
Hoagie or submarine, 11 1/2 by 3 by 2 1/2 in	1 roll	135	390	12	4	.9	75
From home recipe:							
Cloverleaf, 2 1/2-in diam., 2 in high..................................	1 roll	35	120	3	3	.8	20
Spaghetti, enriched, cooked:							
Firm stage, "al dente," served hot...	1 cup	130	190	7	1	—	39
Tender stage, served hot...........	1 cup	140	155	5	1	—	32
Spaghetti (enriched) in tomato sauce with cheese:							
From home recipe......................	1 cup	250	260	9	9	2.0	37
Canned	1 cup	250	190	6	2	.5	39
Spagetti (enriched) with meat balls and tomato sauce:							
From home recipe......................	1 cup	248	330	19	12	3.3	39
Canned	1 cup	250	260	12	10	2.2	29
Toaster pasteries	1 pastry ..	50	200	3	6	—	36
Waffles, made with enriched flour, 7-in diam.:[20]							
From home recipe......................	1 waffle ..	75	210	7	7	2.3	28
From mix, egg and milk added	1 waffle ..	75	205	7	8	2.8	27
Wheat flours:							
All-purpose family flour, enriched:							
Sifted, spooned	1 cup	115	420	12	1	0.2	88
Unsifted, spooned..................	1 cup	125	455	13	1	.2	95
Cake or pastry flour, enriched, sifted, spooned	1 cup	96	350	7	1	.1	76
Self-rising, enriched, unsifted, spooned....................................	1 cup	125	440	12	1	.2	93
Whole-wheat, from hard wheats, stirred	1 cup	120	400	16	2	.4	85

LEGUMES (DRY), NUTS, SEEDS; RELATED PRODUCTS

Almonds, shelled:							
Chopped (about 130 almonds)..	1 cup	130	775	24	70	5.6	25
Slivered, not pressed down (about 15 almonds)...................	1 cup	115	690	21	62	5.0	22
Beans, dry:							
Common varieties as Great Northern, navy, and others:							
Cooked, drained:							

GRAIN PRODUCTS		Grams	Food energy Calories	Protein Grams	Total Fat Grams	Fatty Acids Saturated Grams	Carbohydrate Grams
Great Northern	1 cup	180	210	14	1	—	38
Pea (navy)	1 cup	190	225	15	1	—	40
Canned, solid and liquid:							
White with—							
Frankfurters (sliced)	1 cup	255	365	19	18	—	32
Pork and tomato sauce	1 cup	255	310	16	7	2.4	48
Pork and sweet sauce	1 cup	255	385	16	12	4.3	54
Red kidney	1 cup	255	230	15	1	—	42
Lima, cooked, drained	1 cup	190	260	16	1	—	49
Blackeye peas, dry, cooked (with residual cooking liquid)	1 cup	250	190	13	1	—	35
Brazil nuts, shelled (6-8 large kernels)	1 oz	28	185	4	19	4.8	3
Cashew nuts, roasted in oil	1 cup	140	785	24	64	12.9	41
Coconut meat, fresh:							
Piece, about 2 by 2 by 1/2 in	1 piece	45	155	2	16	14.0	4
Shredded or grated, not pressed down	1 cup	80	275	3	28	24.8	8
Filberts (hazelnuts), chopped (about 80 kernels	1 cup	115	730	14	72	5.1	19
Lentils, whole, cooked	1 cup	200	210	16	Trace	—	39
Peanuts, rosted in oil, salted (whole, halves, chopped)	1 cup	144	840	37	72	13.7	27
Peanut butter	1 tbsp	16	95	4	3	1.5	8
Peas, split, dry, cooked	1 cup	200	230	16	1	—	42
Pecans, chopped or pieces (about 120 large halves)	1 cup	118	810	11	84	7.2	17
Pumpkin and squash kernels, dry, hulled	1 cup	140	775	41	65	11.8	21
Sunflower seeds, dry, hulled	1 cup	145	810	35	69	8.2	29
Walnuts:							
Black:							
Chopped or broken kernels	1 cup	125	785	26	74	6.3	19
Ground (finely)	1 cup	80	500	16	47	4.0	12
Persian or English, chopped (about 60 halves)	1 cup	120	780	18	77	8.4	19
SUGARS AND SWEETS							
Cake icings:							
Boiled, white:							
Plain	1 cup	94	295	1	0	0	75
With coconut	1 cup	166	605	3	13	11.0	124

Uncooked:							
Chocolate made with milk and butter	1 cup	275	1,035	9	38	23.4	185
Creamy fudge from mix and water	1 cup	245	830	7	16	5.1	183
White	1 cup	319	1,200	2	21	12.7	260
Candy:							
Carmels, plain or chocolate	1 oz	28	115	1	3	1.6	22
Chocolate:							
Milk, plain	1 oz	28	145	2	9	5.5	16
Semisweet, small pieces (60 per oz)	1 cup or 6-oz pkg	170	860	7	61	36.2	97
Chocolate-coated peanuts	1 oz	28	160	5	12	4.0	11
Fondant, uncoated (mints, candy corn, other)	1 oz	28	105	Trace	1	.1	25
Fudge, chocolate, plain	1 oz	28	115	1	3	1.3	21
Gum drops	1 oz	28	100	Trace	Trace	—	25
Hard	1 oz	28	110	0	Trace	—	28
Marshmallows	1 oz	28	90	1	Trace	—	23
Chocolate-flavored beverage powders (about 4 heaping tsp per oz):							
With nonfat dry milk	1 oz	28	100	5	1	.5	20
Without milk	1 oz	28	100	1	1	.4	25
Honey, strained or extracted	1 tbsp	21	65	Trace	0	0	17
Jams and preserves	1 tbsp	20	55	Trace	Trace	—	14
	1 packet	14	40	Trace	Trace	—	10
Jellies	1 tbsp	18	50	Trace	Trace	—	13
	1 packet	14	40	Trace	Trace	—	10
Sirups:							
Chocolate-flavored sirup or topping:							
Thin type	1 fl oz or 2 tbsp	38	90	1	1	.5	24
Fudge type	1 fl oz or 2 tbsp	38	125	2	5	3.1	20
Molasses, cane:							
Light (first extraction)	1 tbsp	20	50	—	—	—	13
Blackstrap (third extraction)	1 tbsp	20	45	—	—	—	11
Sorghum	1 tbsp	21	55	—	—	—	14
Table blends, chiefly corn, light and dark	1 tbsp	21	60	0	0	0	15
Sugars:							
Brown, pressed down	1 cup	220	820	0	0	0	212
White:							
Granulated	1 cup	200	770	0	0	0	199
	1 tbsp	12	45	0	0	0	12
	1 packet	6	23	0	0	0	6
Powdered, sifted, spooned into cup	1 cup	100	385	0	0	0	100

VEGETABLES AND VEGETABLE PRODUCTS		Grams	Food energy Calories	Protein Grams	Total Fat Grams	Fatty Acids Saturated Grams	Carbo-hydrate Grams
Asparagus, green:							
Cooked, drained:							
Cuts and tips, 1 1/2- to 2-in lengths:							
From raw	1 cup	145	30	3	Trace	—	5
From frozen	1 cup	180	40	6	Trace	—	6
Spears, 1/2-in diam. at base:							
From raw	4 spears	60	10	1	Trace	—	2
From frozen	4 spears	60	15	2	Trace	—	2
Canned, spears, 1/2-in diam. at base	4 spears	80	15	2	Trace	—	3
Beans:							
Lima, immature seeds, frozen, cooked drained:							
Thick-seeded types (Fordhooks)	1 cup	170	170	10	Trace	—	32
Thin-seeded types (baby limas)	1 cup	180	210	13	Trace	—	40
Snap:							
Green:							
Cooked, drained:							
From raw (cuts and French style)	1 cup	125	30	2	Trace	—	7
From frozen:							
Cuts	1 cup	135	35	2	Trace	—	8
French style	1 cup	130	35	2	Trace	—	8
Canned, drained solids (cuts)	1 cup	135	30	2	Trace	—	7
Yellow or wax:							
Cooked, drained:							
From raw (cuts and French style)	1 cup	125	30	2	Trace	—	6
From frozen (cuts)	1 cup	135	35	2	Trace	—	8
Canned, drained solids (cuts)	1 cup	135	30	2	Trace	—	7
Beans, mature. See Beans, dry (item 509-515) and Blackeye peas, dry (item 516).							
Bean sprouts (mung):							
Raw	1 cup	105	35	4	Trace	—	7
Cooked, drained	1 cup	125	35	4	Trace	—	7
Beets:							
Cooked, drained, peeled:							
Whole beets, 2-in diam.	2 beets	100	30	1	Trace	—	7
Diced or sliced	1 cup	170	55	2	Trace	—	12
Canned, drained solids:							
Whole beets, small	1 cup	160	60	2	Trace	—	14
Diced or sliced	1 cup	170	65	2	Trace	—	15
Beet greens, leaves and stems, cooked, drained	1 cup	145	25	2	Trace	—	5
Blackeye peas, immature seeds, cooked and drained:							

From raw	1 cup	165	180	13	1	—	30
From frozen	1 cup	170	220	15	1	—	40
Broccoli, cooked, drained:							
From raw:							
Stalk, medium size	1 stalk	180	45	6	1	—	8
Stalks cut into 1/2-in pieces	1 cup	155	40	5	Trace	—	7
From frozen:							
Stalk, 4 1/2 to 5 in long	1 stalk	30	10	1	Trace	—	1
Chopped	1 cup	185	50	5	1	—	9
Brussel sprouts, cooked, drained:							
From raw, 7-8 sprouts (1 1/4- to 1 1/2-in diam.)	1 cup	155	55	7	1	—	10
From frozen	1 cup	155	50	5	Trace	—	10
Cabbage:							
Common varieties:							
Raw:							
Coarsely shredded or sliced	1 cup	70	15	1	Trace	—	4
Finely shredded or chopped	1 cup	90	20	1	Trace	—	5
Cooked, drained	1 cup	145	30	2	Trace	—	6
Red, raw, coarsely shredded or sliced	1 cup	70	20	1	Trace	—	5
Savoy, raw, coarsely shredded or sliced	1 cup	70	15	2	Trace	—	3
Cabbage, celery (also called pe-tsai or wongbok), raw, 1-in pieces	1 cup	75	10	1	Trace	—	2
Cabbage, white mustard (also called bokchoy or pakchoy), cooked, drained.	1 cup	170	25	2	Trace	—	4
Carrots:							
Raw, without crowns and tips, scraped:							
Whole, 7 1/2 by 1 1/8 in, or strips, 2 1/2 to 3 in long	1 carrot or 18 strips	72	30	1	Trace	—	7
Grated	1 cup	110	45	1	Trace	—	11
Cooked (crosswise cuts), drained	1 cup	155	50	1	Trace	—	11
Canned:							
Sliced, drained solids	1 cup	155	45	1	Trace	—	10
Strained or junior (baby food)	1 oz (1 3/4 to 2 tbsp)	28	10	Trace	Trace	—	2
Cauliflower:							
Raw, chopped	1 cup	115	31	3	Trace	—	6
Cooked, drained:							
From raw (flower buds)	1 cup	125	30	3	Trace	—	5
From frozen (flowerets)	1 cup	180	30	3	Trace	—	6

		Grams	Food energy Calories	Protein Grams	Total Fat Grams	Fatty Acids Saturated Grams	Carbo-hydrate Grams
Celery, Pascal type, raw:							
Stalk, large outer, 8 by 1 1/2 in, at root end	1 stalk	40	5	Trace	Trace	—	2
Pieces, diced	1 cup	120	20	1	Trace	—	5
Collards, cooked, drained:							
From raw (leaves without stems)	1 cup	190	65	7	1	—	10
From frozen (chopped)	1 cup	170	50	5	1	—	10
Corn, sweet:							
Cooked, drained:							
From raw, ear 5 by 1 3/4 in	1 ear[31]	140	70	2	1	—	16
From frozen:							
Ear, 5 in long	1 ear[31]	229	120	4	1	—	27
Kernels	1 cup	165	130	5	1	—	31
Canned:							
Cream style	1 cup	256	210	5	2	—	51
Whole kernel:							
Vacuum pack	1 cup	210	175	5	1	—	43
Wet pack, drained solids	1 cup	165	140	4	1	—	33
Cucumber slices, 1/8 in thick (large, 2 1/8-in diam; small, 1 3/4-in diam):							
With peel	6 large or 8 small slices	28	5	Trace	Trace	—	1
Without peel	1 cup	28	5	Trace	Trace	—	1
Dandelion greens, cooked, drained	1 cup	105	35	2	1	—	7
Endive, curly (including escarole), raw, small pieces	1 cup	50	10	1	Trace	—	2
Kale, cooked, drained:							
From raw (leaves without stems and midribs)	1 cup	110	45	5	1	—	7
From frozen (leaf style)	1 cup	130	40	4	1	—	7
Lettuce, raw:							
Butterhead, as Boston types:							
Head, 5-in diam	1 head[32]	220	25	2	Trace	—	4
Leaves	1 outer or 2 inner or 3 heart leaves	15	Trace	Trace	Trace	—	Trace
Crisphead, as Iceberg:							
Head, 6-in diam	1 head[33]	567	70	5	1	—	16
Wedge, 1/4 of head	1 wedge	135	20	1	Trace	—	4
Pieces, chopped or shredded	1 cup	55	5	Trace	Trace	—	2
Looseleaf (bunching varieties including romaine or cos), chopped or shredded pieces	1 cup	55	10	1	Trace	—	2
Mushrooms, raw, sliced or							

chopped	1 cup	70	20	2	Trace	—	3
Mustard greens, without stems and midribs, cooked, drained	1 cup	140	30	3	1	—	6
Okra pods, 3 by 5/8 in, cooked	10 pods	106	30	2	Trace	—	6
Onions:							
Mature:							
Raw:							
Chopped	1 cup	170	65	3	Trace	—	15
Sliced	1 cup	115	45	2	Trace	—	10
Cooked (whole or sliced), drained	1 cup	210	60	3	Trace	—	14
Young green, bulb (3/8 in diam) and white portion of top	6 onions	30	15	Trace	Trace	—	3
Parsley, raw, chopped	1 tbsp	4	Trace	Trace	Trace	—	Trace
Parsnips, cooked (diced or 2-in lengths)	1 cup	155	100	2	1	—	23
Peas, green:							
Canned:							
Whole, drained solids	1 cup	170	150	8	1	—	29
Strained (baby food)	1 oz (1 3/4 to 2 tbsp)	28	15	1	Trace	—	3
Frozen, cooked, drained	1 cup	160	110	8	Trace	—	19
Peppers, hot, red, without seeds, dried, (ground chili powder, added seasonings)	1 tsp	2	5	Trace	Trace	—	1
Peppers, sweet (about 5 per lb, whole), stem and seeds removed:							
Raw	1 pod	74	15	1	Trace	—	4
Cooked, boiled, drained	1 pod	73	15	1	Trace	—	3
Potatoes, cooked:							
Baked, peeled after baking (about 2 per lb, raw)	1 potato	156	145	4	Trace	—	33
Boiled (about 3 per lb, raw):							
Peeled after boiling	1 potato	137	105	3	Trace	—	23
Peeled before boiling	1 potato	135	90	3	Trace	—	20
French-fried, strip, 2 to 3 1/2 in long:							
Prepared from raw	10 strips	50	135	2	7	1.7	18
Frozen, oven heated	10 strips	50	110	2	4	1.1	17
Hashed brown, prepared from frozen	1 cup	155	345	3	18	4.6	45
Mashed, prepared from—							
Raw:							
Milk added	1 cup	210	135	4	2	.7	27
Milk and butter added	1 cup	210	195	4	9	5.6	26
Dehydrated flakes (without milk), water, milk, butter, and salt added	1 cup	210	195	4	7	3.6	30

		Grams	Food energy Calories	Protein Grams	Total Fat Grams	Fatty Acids Saturated Grams	Carbo-hydrate Grams
Potato chips, 1 3/4 by 2 1/2 in oval cross section	10 chips	20	115	1	8	2.1	10
Potato salad, made with cooked salad dressing	1 cup	250	250	7	7	2.0	41
Pumpkin, canned	1 cup	245	80	2	1	—	19
Radishes, raw (prepackaged) stem ends, rootlets cut off	4 radishes	18	5	Trace	Trace	—	1
Sauerkraut, canned, solids and liquid	1 cup	235	40	2	Trace	—	9
Spinach:							
Raw, chopped	1 cup	55	15	2	Trace	—	2
Cooked, drained:							
From raw	1 cup	180	40	5	1	—	6
From frozen:							
Chopped	1 cup	205	45	6	1	—	8
Leaf	1 cup	190	45	6	1	—	7
Canned, drained solids	1 cup	205	50	6	1	—	7
Squash, cooked:							
Summer (all varieties), diced, drained	1 cup	210	30	2	Trace	—	7
Winter (all varieties), baked, mashed	1 cup	205	130	4	1	—	32
Sweetpotatoes:							
Cooked (raw, 5 by 2 in; about 2 1/2 per lb):							
Baked in skin, peeled	1 potato	114	160	2	1	—	37
Boiled in skin, peeled	1 potato	151	170	3	1	—	40
Candied, 2 1/2 by 2-in piece	1 piece	105	175	1	3	2.0	36
Canned:							
Solid pack (mashed)	1 cup	255	275	5	1	—	63
Vacuum pack, piece 2 3/4 by 1 in	1 piece	40	45	1	Trace	—	10
Tomatoes:							
Raw, 2 3/5-in diam (3 per 12 oz pkg)	1 tomato[34]	135	25	1	Trace	—	6
Canned, solids and liquid	1 cup	241	50	2	Trace	—	10
Tomato catsup	1 cup	273	290	5	1	—	69
	1 tbsp	15	15	Trace	Trace	—	4
Tomato juice, canned:							
Cup	1 cup	243	45	2	Trace	—	10
Glass (6 fl oz)	1 glass	182	35	2	Trace	—	8
Turnips, cooked, diced	1 cup	155	35	1	Trace	—	8
Turnip greens, cooked, drained:							
From raw (leaves and stems)	1 cup	145	30	3	Trace	—	5

From frozen (chopped)	1 cup	165	40	4	Trace	—	6
Vegetables, mixed, frozen, cooked	1 cup	182	115	6	1	—	24

MISCELLANEOUS ITEMS

Baking powders for home use:							
Sodium aluminum sulfate:							
With monocalcium phosphate monohydrate	1 tsp	3.0	5	Trace	Trace	0	1
With monocalcium phosphate monohydrate, calcium sulfate	1 tsp	2.9	5	Trace	Trace	0	1
Straight phosphate	1 tsp	3.8	5	Trace	Trace	0	1
Low sodium	1 tsp	4.3	5	Trace	Trace	0	2
Barbecue sauce	1 cup	250	230	4	17	2.2	20
Beverages, alcoholic:							
Beer	12 fl oz	360	150	1	0	0	14
Gin, rum, vodka, whisky:							
80-proof	1 1/2-fl oz jigger	42	95	—	—	0	Trace
86-proof	1 1/2-fl oz jigger	42	105	—	—	0	Trace
90-proof	1 1/2-fl oz jigger	42	110	—	—	0	Trace
Wines:							
Dessert	3 1/2-fl oz glass	103	140	Trace	0	0	8
Table	3 1/2-fl oz glass	102	85	Trace	0	0	4
Beverages, carbonated, sweetened, nonalcoholic:							
Carbonated water	12 fl oz	366	115	0	0	0	29
Cola type	12 fl oz	369	145	0	0	0	37
Fruit-flavored sodas and Tom Collins mixer	12 fl oz	372	170	0	0	0	45
Ginger ale	12 fl oz	366	115	0	0	0	29
Root beer	12 fl oz	370	150	0	0	0	39
Chocolate:							
Bitter or baking	1 oz	28	145	3	15	8.9	8
Gelatin, dry	1.7-g envelope	7	25	6	Trace	0	0
Gelatin dessert prepared with gelatin dessert powder and water	1 cup	240	140	4	0	0	34
Mustard, prepared, yellow	1 tsp or individual serving 5 pouch or cup	5	5	Trace	Trace	—	Trace

		Grams	Food energy Calories	Protein Grams	Total Fat Grams	Fatty Acids Saturated Grams	Carbo-hydrate Grams
Olives, pickled, canned:							
Green	4 medium or 3 extra large or 2 giant[35]	16	15	Trace	2	.2	Trace
Ripe, Mission	3 small or 2 large[35]	10	15	Trace	2	.2	Trace
Pickles, cucumber:							
Dill, medium, whole, 3 3/4 in long, 1 1/4-in diam	1 pickle	65	5	Trace	Trace	—	1
Fresh-pack, slices 1 1/2-in diam, 1/4 in thick	2 slices	15	10	Trace	Trace	—	3
Sweet, gherkin, small, whole, about 2 1/2 in long, 3/4-in diam	1 pickle	15	20	Trace	Trace	—	5
Relish, finely chopped, sweet	1 tbsp	15	20	Trace	Trace	—	5
Popsicle, 3-fl oz size	1 popsicle	95	70	0	0	0	18
Soups:							
Canned, condensed:							
Prepared with equal volume of milk:							
Cream of chicken	1 cup	245	180	7	10	4.2	15
Cream of mushroom	1 cup	245	215	7	14	5.4	16
Tomato	1 cup	250	175	7	7	3.4	23
Prepared with equal volume of water:							
Bean with pork	1 cup	250	170	8	6	1.2	22
Beef broth, bouillon, consomme	1 cup	240	30	5	0	0	3
Beef noodle	1 cup	240	65	4	3	.6	7
Clam chowder, Manhattan type (with tomatoes, without milk)	1 cup	245	80	2	3	.5	12
Cream of chicken	1 cup	240	95	3	6	1.6	8
Cream of mushroom	1 cup	240	135	2	10	2.6	10
Minestrone	1 cup	245	105	5	3	.7	14
Split pea	1 cup	245	145	9	3	1.1	21
Tomato	1 cup	245	90	2	3	.5	16
Vegetable beef	1 cup	245	80	5	2	—	10
Vegetarian	1 cup	245	80	2	2	—	13
Dehydrated:							
Bouillon cube, 1/2 in	1 cube	4	5	1	Trace	—	Trace
Mixes:							
Unprepared:							
Onion	1 1/2-oz pkg	43	150	6	5	1.1	23
Prepared with water:							
Chicken noodle	1 cup	240	55	2	1	—	8
Onion	1 cup	240	35	1	1	—	6
Tomato vegetable with noodles	1 cup	240	65	1	1	—	12
Vinegar, cider	1 tbsp	15	Trace	Trace	0	0	1

White sauce, medium, with enriched flour	1 cup	250	405	10	31	19.3	22
Yeast:							
Baker's, dry, active	1 pkg	7	20	3	Trace	—	3
Brewer's, dry	1 tbsp	8	25	3	Trace	—	3

[1] Yields 1 qt of fluid milk when reconstituted according to package directions.
[2] Weight applies to product with label claim of 1 1/3 cups equal 3.2 oz.
[3] Applies to products made from thick shake mixes and that do not contain added ice cream. Products made from milk shake mixes are higher in fat and usually contain added ice cream.
[4] Fatty acid values apply to product made with regular-type margarine.
[5] Dipped in egg, milk or water, and breadcrumbs; fried in vegetable shortening.
[6] Dipped in egg, breadcrumbs, and flour or batter.
[7] Prepared with tuna, celery, salad dressing (mayonnaise type), pickle, onion, and egg.
[8] Outer layer of fat on the cut was removed to within approximately 1/2 in of the lean. Deposits of fat within the cut were not removed.
[9] Crust made with vegetable shortening and enriched flour.
[10] Regular-type margarine used.
[11] About one-fourth of the outer layer of fat on the cut was removed. Deposits of fat within the cut were not removed.
[12] Vegetable shortening used.
[13] Also applies to pasteurized apple cider.
[14] Weight includes peel and membranes between sections.
[15] For white-fleshed varieties, value is about 20 International Units (I.U.) per cup; for red-fleshed varieties, 1,080 I.U.
[16] Weight includes seeds.
[17] Weight includes rind. Without rind, the weight of the edible portion is 272 g for item 271 and 149 g for item 272.
[18] Weight includes pits.
[19] Weight includes rind and seeds. Without rind and seeds, weight of the edible portion is 426 g.
[20] Made with vegetable shortening.
[21] Applies to product made with white cornmeal. With yellow cornmeal, value is 30 International Units (I.U.).
[22] Applies to white varieties. For yellow varieties, value is 150 International Units (I.U.).
[23] Applies to products that do not contain di-sodium phosphate. If di-sodium phosphate is an ingredient, value is 162 mg.
[24] Value may range from less than 1 mg to about 8 mg depending on the brand. Consult the label.
[25] Excepting angelfood cake, cakes were made from mixes containing vegetable shortening; icings, with butter.
[26] Equal weights of flour, sugar, eggs, and vegetable shortening.
[27] Products are commercial unless otherwise specified.
[28] Made with enriched flour and vegetable shortening except for macaroons which do not contain flour or shortening.
[29] Made with vegetable shortening.
[30] Products are commercial unless otherwise specified.
[31] Made with enriched flour and vegetable shortening except for macaroons which do not contain flour or shortening.
[32] Contains vegetable shortening and butter.
[33] Made with corn oil.
[34] Made with regular margarine.
[35] Made with enriched degermed cornmeal and enriched flour.
[36] Weight includes cob. Without cob, weight is 77 g for item 612, 126 g for item 613.
[37] Weight includes refuse of outer leaves and core. Without these parts, weight is 163 g.
[38] Weight includes core. Without core, weight is 539 g.
[39] Weight includes cores and stem ends. Without these parts, weight is 123 g.
[40] Weight includes pits. Without pits, weight is 13 g for item 701, 9 g for item 702.

Source: Home and Garden Bulletin No. 72 (Rev. 1977) United States Department of Agriculture

1983 METROPOLITAN HEIGHT AND WEIGHT TABLES FOR MEN AND WOMEN

According to Frame, Ages 25–59

HEIGHT (In Shoes)†		Weight in Pounds (In Indoor Clothing)*		
		SMALL FRAME	MEDIUM FRAME	LARGE FRAME
Feet	Inches		MEN	
5	2	128–134	131–141	138–150
5	3	130–136	133–143	140–153
5	4	132–138	135–145	142–156
5	5	134–140	137–148	144–160
5	6	136–142	139–151	146–164
5	7	138–145	142–154	149–168
5	8	140–148	145–157	152–172
5	9	142–151	148–160	155–176
5	10	144–154	151–163	158–180
5	11	146–157	154–166	161–184
6	0	149–160	157–170	164–188
6	1	152–164	160–174	168–192
6	2	155–168	164–178	172–197
6	3	158–172	167–182	176–202
6	4	162–176	171–187	181–207
			WOMEN	
4	10	102–111	109–121	118–131
4	11	103–113	111–123	120–134
5	0	104–115	113–126	122–137
5	1	106–118	115–129	125–140
5	2	108–121	118–132	128–143
5	3	111–124	121–135	131–147
5	4	114–127	124–138	134–151
5	5	117–130	127–141	137–155
5	6	120–133	130–144	140–159
5	7	123–136	133–147	143–163
5	8	126–139	136–150	146–167
5	9	129–142	139–153	149–170
5	10	132–145	142–156	152–173
5	11	135–148	145–159	155–176
6	0	138–151	148–162	158–179

*Indoor clothing weighing 5 pounds for men and 3 pounds for women.
†Shoes with 1-inch heels.

HOW TO DETERMINE YOUR BODY FRAME BY ELBOW BREADTH

To make a simple approximation of your frame size:

Extend your arm and bend the forearm upwards at a 90-degree angle. Keep the fingers straight and turn the inside of your wrist toward the body. Place the thumb and index finger of your other hand on the two prominent bones on either side of your elbow. Measure the space between your fingers against a ruler or a tape measure. (For the most accurate measurement, have your physician measure your elbow breadth with calipers.) Compare this measurement with the measurements shown below.

These tables list the elbow measurements for men and women of medium frame at various heights. Measurements lower than those listed indicate that you have a small frame while higher measurements indicate a large frame.

MEN

HEIGHT (In 1-inch Heels)	ELBOW BREADTH (Inches)	HEIGHT (In 2.3-cm. Heels)	ELBOW BREADTH (Centimeters)
5′2″–5′3″	2 1/2″–2 7/8″	158–161	6.4–7.2
5′4″–5′7″	2 5/8″–2 7/8″	162–171	6.7–7.4
5′8″–5′11″	2 3/4″–3″	172–181	6.9–7.6
6′0″–6′3″	2 3/4″–3 1/8″	182–191	7.1–7.8
6′4″	2 7/8″–3 1/4″	192–193	7.4–8.1

WOMEN

HEIGHT (In 1-inch Heels)	ELBOW BREADTH (Inches)	HEIGHT (In 2.5-cm. Heels)	ELBOW BREADTH (Centimeters)
4′10″–4′11″	2 1/4″–2 1/2″	148–151	5.6–6.4
5′0″–5′3″	2 1/4″–2 1/2″	152–161	5.8–6.5
5′4″–5′7″	2 3/8″–2 5/8″	162–171	5.9–6.6
5′8″–5′11″	2 3/8″–2 5/8″	172–181	6.1–6.8
6′0″	2 1/2″–2 3/4″	182–183	6.2–6.9

FOOD AND NUTRITION BOARD, NATIONAL ACADEMY OF SCIENCES—NATIONAL RESEARCH COUNCIL RECOMMENDED DAILY DIETARY ALLOWANCES,[a] Revised 1980

Designed for the maintenance of good nutrition of practically all healthy people in the U.S.A.

FAT-SOLUBLE VITAMINS

	Age (years)	Weight (lb)	Height (in)	Protein (g)	Vitamin A (μg RE)[b]	Vitamin D (μg)[f]	Vitamin E (mg α-TE)[d]
Infants	0.0–0.5	13	24	kg × 2.2	420	10	3
	0.5–1.0	20	28	kg × 2.0	400	10	4
Children	1–3	29	35	23	400	10	5
	4–6	44	44	30	500	10	6
	7–10	62	52	34	700	10	7
Males	11–14	99	62	45	1000	10	8
	15–18	145	69	56	1000	10	10
	19–22	154	70	56	1000	7.5	10
	23–50	154	70	56	1000	5	10
	51+	154	70	56	1000	5	10
Females	11–14	101	62	46	800	10	8
	15–18	120	64	46	800	10	8
	19–22	120	64	44	800	7.5	8
	23–50	120	64	44	800	5	8
	51+	120	64	44	800	5	8
Pregnant				+30	+200	+5	+2
Lactating				+20	+400	+5	+3

WATER-SOLUBLE VITAMINS

	Age (years)	Weight (lb)	Height (in)	Vitamin C (mg)	Thiamin (mg)	Riboflavin (mg)	Niacin (mg NE)[c]	Vitamin B-6 (mg)	Folacin[f] (μg)	Vitamin B-12 (μg)
Infants	0.0–0.5	13	24	35	0.3	0.4	6	0.3	30	0.5[g]
	0.5–1.0	20	28	35	0.5	0.6	8	0.6	45	1.5[g]
Children	1–3	29	35	45	0.7	0.8	9	0.9	100	2.0
	4–6	44	44	45	0.9	1.0	11	1.3	200	2.5
	7–10	62	52	45	1.2	1.4	16	1.6	300	3.0
Males	11–14	99	62	50	1.4	1.6	18	1.8	400	3.0
	15–18	145	69	60	1.4	1.7	18	2.0	400	3.0
	19–22	154	70	60	1.5	1.7	19	2.2	400	3.0
	23–50	154	70	60	1.4	1.6	18	2.2	400	3.0
	51+	154	70	60	1.2	1.4	16	2.2	400	3.0
Females	11–14	101	62	50	1.1	1.3	15	1.8	400	3.0
	15–18	120	64	60	1.1	1.3	14	2.0	400	3.0
	19–22	120	64	60	1.1	1.3	14	2.0	400	3.0
	23–50	120	64	60	1.0	1.2	13	2.0	400	3.0
	51+	120	64	60	1.0	1.2	13	2.0	400	3.0
Pregnant				+20	+0.4	+0.3	+2	+0.6	+400	+1.0
Lactating				+40	+0.5	+0.5	+5	+0.5	+100	+1.0

MINERALS

	Age (years)	Weight (lb)	Height (in)	Calcium (mg)	Phosphorus (mg)	Magnesium (mg)	Iron (mg)	Zinc (mg)	Iodine (μg)
Infants	0.0–0.5	13	24	360	240	50	10	3	40
	0.5–1.0	20	28	540	360	70	15	5	50
Children	1–3	29	35	800	800	150	15	10	70
	4–6	44	44	800	800	200	10	10	90
	7–10	62	52	800	800	250	10	10	120
Males	11–14	99	62	1200	1200	350	18	15	150
	15–18	145	69	1200	1200	400	18	15	150
	19–22	154	70	800	800	350	10	10	150
	23–50	154	70	800	800	350	10	15	150
	51+	154	70	800	800	350	10	15	150
Females	11–14	101	62	1200	1200	300	18	15	150
	15–18	120	64	1200	1200	300	18	15	150
	19–22	120	64	800	800	300	18	15	150
	23–50	120	64	800	800	300	18	15	150
	51+	120	64	800	800	300	10	15	150
Pregnant				+400	+400	+150	[h]	+5	+25
Lactating				+400	+400	+150	[h]	+10	+50

Daily Calories Average Weights at Average Heights[a]

Category	Age (years)	WEIGHT (lb)	HEIGHT (in)	ENERGY NEEDS (kcal)
Children	1–3	29	35	1300
	4–6	44	44	1700
	7–10	62	52	2400
Males	11–14	99	62	2700
	15–18	145	69	2800
	19–22	154	70	2900
	23–50	154	70	2700
	51–75	154	70	2400
	76+	154	70	2050
Females	11–14	101	62	2200
	15–18	120	64	2100
	19–22	120	64	2100
	23–50	120	64	2000
	51–75	120	64	1800
	76+	120	64	1600
Pregnancy				+300
Lactation				+500

Source: National Academy of Sciences

Estimated Safe and Adequate Daily Dietary Intakes of Selected Vitamins and Minerals[a]

VITAMINS

	Age (years)	Vitamin K (μg)	Biotin (μg)	Pantothenic Acid (mg)
Infants	0–0.5	12	35	2
	0.5–1	10–20	50	3
Children	1–3	15–30	65	3
and	4–6	20–40	85	3–4
Adolescents	7–10	30–60	120	4–5
	11+	50–100	100–200	4–7
Adults		70–140	100–200	4–7

TRACE ELEMENTS[b]

	Age (years)	Copper (mg)	Manganese (mg)	Fluoride (mg)	Chromium (mg)	Selenium (mg)	Molybdenum (mg)
Infants	0–0.5	0.5–0.7	0.5–0.7	0.1–0.5	0.01–0.04	0.01–0.04	0.03–0.06
	0.5–1	0.7–1.0	0.7–1.0	0.2–1.0	0.02–0.06	0.02–0.06	0.04–0.08
Children	1–3	1.0–1.5	1.0–1.5	0.5–1.5	0.02–0.08	0.02–0.08	0.05–0.1
and	4–6	1.5–2.0	1.5–2.0	1.0–2.5	0.03–0.12	0.03–0.12	0.06–0.15
Adolescents	7–10	2.0–2.5	2.0–3.0	1.5–2.5	0.05–0.2	0.05–0.2	0.10–0.3
	11+	2.0–3.0	2.5–5.0	1.5–2.5	0.05–0.2	0.05–0.2	0.15–0.5
Adults		2.0–3.0	2.5–5.0	1.5–4.0	0.05–0.2	0.05–0.2	0.15–0.5

ELECTROLYTES

	Age (years)	Sodium (mg)	Potassium (mg)	Chloride (mg)
Infants	0–0.5	115–350	350–925	275–700
	0.5–1	250–750	425–1275	400–1200
Children	1–3	325–975	550–1650	500–1500
and	4–6	450–1350	775–2325	700–2100
Adolescents	7–10	600–1800	1000–3000	925–2775
	11+	900–2700	1525–4575	1400–4200
Adults		1100–3300	1875–5625	1700–5100

INDEX

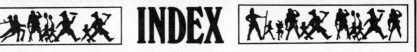

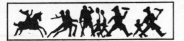